Animal Medicines
A User's Guide

This booklet is, in effect, the third version of 'The Safe Storage and Handling of Animal Medicines' originally produced by the Association of the British Pharmaceutical Industry (ABPI) in 1982 and revised by NOAH in 1990.

Every effort has been made to ensure that the information contained herein is accurate as at October 1995. However, neither NOAH nor the authors can accept any responsibility for the information provided. Legislation may change considerably in the next few years.

ISBN: 0 9526638 2 1

Published by National Office of Animal Health Ltd.
3 Crossfield Chambers, Gladbeck Way, Enfield EN2 7HF
Printed by Reprodux Printers, Station Approach, Commercial Road, Hereford, HR1 1BB

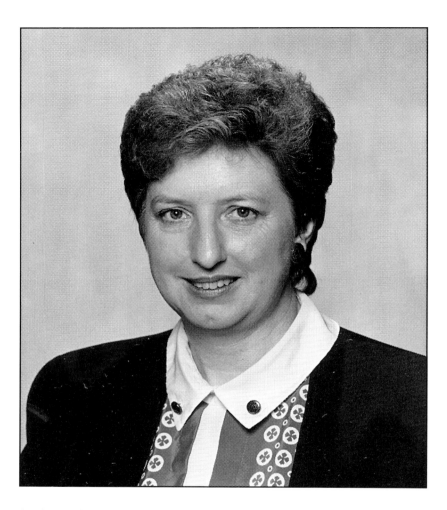

Angela Browning, MP
Parliamentary Secretary, Ministry of Agriculture, Fisheries and Food

Foreword

By the Parliamentary Secretary, Ministry of Agriculture, Fisheries and Food

It is vital that those who handle animal medicines in their day-to-day work on farms are well-informed about the potential risks involved. All animal medicines must be treated with proper respect for the potential risks to the animal, the operator and the environment. This is particularly the case for ectoparasiticides which depend for their efficacy on their toxic properties.

No animal medicine is authorised for the market until it has undergone the most rigorous examination for safety, quality and efficacy. But in the end, it is the people handling and using the product who must make judgements based on advice and label requirements.

It is important to have a full understanding of how to handle, store and transport these products. For this reason, NOAH are to be commended for producing such a succinct and helpful booklet for the farming industry and agricultural supply trades. As usual, it includes a review of current legislation and changes, complementing information available from the Veterinary Medicines Directorate.

This compendium of valuable advice can be thoroughly recommended to all those responsible for the storage, handling and supply of animal medicines.

Angela Browning MP

Contents

	Foreword	*Angela Browning MP*	3
	Introduction	*Richard Crow*	5
1.	Legal Requirements Governing the Distribution of Animal Medicines	*C C Stevens revised by Gordon E Applebe*	6
2.	Controlled Drugs	*W Derek Tavernor*	12
3.	Health & Safety at Work, etc Act 1974	*R E Ablett revised by Cameron N Downie*	24
4.	Implementation of COSHH Legislation on Industry	*Cameron N Downie*	31
5.	Storage, Transportation & Aspects of Safety in Veterinary Practice	*J Tandy revised by Bas D W Hardy*	39
6.	Transport of Animal Medicines	*Roger R Cook & Stephen Dawson*	47
7.	Dispensing, Labelling & Manufacturers Instructions	*P D Simm revised by Michael H Jepson*	52
8.	Sterility & Sterile Products	*J E Brown revised by John Dowrick*	63
9.	Antibiotics	*A B Marshall revised by Robin Bywater*	67
10.	Vaccines	*A S H Miller revised by Gillian Cowan*	72
11.	Antiparasitic Products	*Peter D G Bowen*	78
12.	Medicinal Feed Additives	*David R Williams*	86
13.	Use of Medicines on Farms	*Roger R Cook*	92
14.	Protection of the Consumer	*Kevin N Woodward*	99
15.	Disposal of Animal Medicines	*Roger R Cook*	105
	Appendix		110

Introduction

Richard Crow, NOAH Public Affairs Committee Chairman

The route from discovery through development and registration for a new animal medicine is tortuous to say the least. It is estimated that only about 1 in 10,000 compounds which are synthesized actually make the grade as a fully licensed product, the remaining 9,999 faltering along the way due to unacceptable efficacy, safety or quality and even manufacturing difficulties.

That 1 product in 10,000 is therefore of great value and with the ever increasing stringency and costs of the licensing procedure, is becoming more and more difficult to find.

The importance of animal medicines for the relief of suffering and production of wholesome meat has never been in question; the world as a whole would be a poorer, sadder place without them. However it should not be forgotten that their use is coming under every closer scrutiny as consumer fears of misuse and residues, abuse and animal welfare are fired by the proliferation of media half-truths and by very rare cases of irresponsible malpractice, which are assumed to be the norm.

So those who are involved in any way with the storage and handling of animal medicines, be they farmers, veterinary surgeons, pharmacists, agricultural merchants or even the general public, must appreciate that they have in their care products, which when treated appropriately are a potent force for the good of both animal and man, but if they are abused the converse can also be true.

This booklet is intended to supplement the specific information contained on product labels, package inserts or data sheets, providing an easy to read guide to legislation relating to medicine storage and handling as well as offering solid advice based on science, common sense and the wealth of experience gained over the years by the contributing authors.

It is a 'must' for keeping within easy reach of all involved in the storage and handling of animal medicines.

Chapter 1

Legal Requirements Governing the Distribution of Animal Medicines

C C Stevens revised by Gordon E Applebe

The legal requirements covering the distribution of animal medicines differ according to the legal classification of the individual product. The classification determines who may sell the product and under what restraint or control. All medicines fall within one or more of the following categories:

Controlled drugs
Specially restricted products such as narcotics and habit forming drugs (See Chapter 2).

Prescription only medicines (POM)
Can be supplied only by a veterinarian for administration to animals under his care or by a pharmacist on the authority of a prescription written by a veterinarian[1].

Pharmacist only medicines (P)
Supplied over the counter for registered pharmacies; and by veterinarians for administration to animals under his care[2].

Merchants list (PML)
Specially listed veterinary products that can be supplied by veterinarians to those having animals under the treatment or control of the veterinarian and over the counter by pharmacists and registered animal health distributors to any person who keeps or maintains animals for the purpose of carrying on a business[3].

Saddlers list
PML products on a short list of horse wormers that may be sold by registered saddlers to horse owners or those having care of horses. These products may also be sold by merchants additionally registering for such purpose at no extra charge. Pharmacists may also sell horse wormers.

General sale list (GSL)
Products that may be sold over the counter by anyone, or from any place[4].

The lists are long and complicated and include variations and exemptions depending upon the dosage, indications or strengths of the active ingredients. Labelling regulations require Prescription Only products to be labelled "POM", Pharmacy only "P", Merchants and Saddlers Lists "PML" and General Sales List "GSL". Manufacturers will label accordingly but vendors should not rely on that alone to guide them upon classification. Distributors may consult the publication "Medicines and Poisons Guide" published by the Royal Pharmaceutical Society of Great Britain, 1 Lambeth High Street, London which in addition to giving useful information on classification and labelling, lists all the medicines, generic and proprietary, human and veterinary, with a clear indication of the lists into which they fall. The lists and the requirements in each case are described below.

Controlled Drugs

These may be supplied by a veterinarian or by a pharmacist on a veterinarian's prescription. The requirements are specific. Controlled Drugs are dealt with fully in Chapter 2.

Prescription only medicines (POM)

These may be supplied by a veterinarian for administration to animals under his care or by a registered pharmacy on a veterinarian's prescription. The prescription must:

a)   be written in indelible ink
b)   contain the following particulars:
      i)   the address and usual signature of the veterinarian
      ii)   the date on which it was signed by the veterinarian
      iii)   an indication that the writer is a veterinary surgeon or a veterinary practitioner
      iv)   the name and address of the person to whom the medicine is to be delivered
(c)   not be dispensed later than six months from the date on it

The pharmacist must keep a record of every sale or supply of a POM. These records must be preserved for two years from the date of the last entry in the register. The details to be recorded are:

a)   the date on which the medicines are sold or supplied
b)   the name and quantity and, where not obvious, the form and strength of the medicine
c)   the date on the prescription and the name and address of the veterinarian that signed it
d)   the name and address of the person for whose animal the medicine was prescribed

Pharmacy only medicines (P)
These may be supplied by a veterinarian for administration to animals under his care or a registered pharmacy. When supplied from a pharmacy, the sale, or supply must be made under the supervision of a pharmacist. This is interpreted in law as being within sight and hearing of the pharmacist. If the supply is handled by an unqualified person, the pharmacist must be able to intervene, if necessary.

The storage of POM and P medicines at the pharmacy is governed by the RPSGB Code of Ethics available from RPSGB.

Merchants list products (PML)
These may be sold by veterinarians to clients having animals under the control of the veterinarian, and from registered pharmacies to any customer. No records are necessary and pharmacies may sell over the counter without supervision. Registered animal health distributors are allowed to sell PML products subject to a number of stringent conditions, the details of which are:

a) they must be persons carrying on a business wholly or mainly comprising the sale by retail of veterinary drugs and other agricultural requisites

b) the trader, before selling, must register with the Royal Pharmaceutical Society (in Northern Ireland - the Department of Agriculture) the location of the premises which must be of a permanent nature. No van sales of PML products are allowed. The Society may satisfy itself as to compliance with the law and undertakings to adhere to the merchants' code of practice before registration. A registration fee and thereafter an annual fee for continuing on the register is payable. Each set of premises must have a nominated person who is responsible for observance of the law and code. A list of acceptably qualified or experienced nominated persons is kept by the Animal Medicines Training and Regulatory Authority (AMTRA), 8 Parsons Hill, Hollesley, Woodbridge, Suffolk. The premises must be occupied and under the control of the seller at the time of the sale and they must be capable of excluding the general public.

The premises must be:

a) a building or part of a building of a permanent nature, or
b) a stall or other similar structure of a permanent nature, situated at a market or agricultural show ground.

The conditions of sale are:

a) the product must be in original unopened containers (pharmacists and veterinarians by contrast may break bulk).
b) the sale must be made to a person whom the seller knows or has reasonable cause to believe is a person in charge of, or maintaining, animals as a part of his business.
c) the product must be in the form set out in the Merchants List, labelled in strength, and dose, together with any special requirements set out in the Schedule to the Order governing these products. As only original packs can be sold by distributors these matters are the concern of the manufacturer. The distributor can assume, when he received the products, that they are labelled and packed properly.
d) Records must be kept of every sale, the date of sale, name, quantity, form, strength of product, and name and address of the purchaser. An invoice or order will suffice in place of a formal register. All records must be kept for two years.

Storage

Animal health distributors must store PML products as set out in the instructions on labels and leaflets. The goods must be out of reach of the public and not sold by self-service methods. The regulations stipulate that they must be "partitioned off and otherwise separate from other parts of the premises to which the public has access".

Saddlers list products (PML)

A short list of horse wormers that may be sold by registered saddlers to horse owners or keepers. Registration is with the Royal Pharmaceutical Society and conditions are similar to those applying to animal health distributors. The saddlers list is now a permanent feature of the legislation and in addition to practising saddlers already registered, new ones must have a nominated person (qualified to AMTRA or British Equestrian Trade Association (BETA) standards).

General sale list products (GSL)

These can be sold by anyone. There is no registration and no special controls on the retailer although wholesalers must be registered. They must be sold, other than by veterinarians or pharmacists, in original and unbroken packs.

Veterinary drugs incorporated in animal feeding stuffs

a) A veterinary surgeon may prescribe, in the form of a veterinary written direction (VWD) or supply any drug for incorporation in feeding stuffs,

provided that the animals for which they are intended, are under his professional care.
b) A pharmacy may dispense a veterinary surgeon's prescription for such drugs. A number of drugs specially designated in the medicines (Exemptions from Restrictions on the Retail Sale or Supply of Veterinary Drugs) Order may be supplied without a prescription.
c) There are special conditions for those who are not veterinarians or pharmacists. The unqualified person must be one carrying on a business wholly or mainly comprising either the manufacture of animal feeding stuffs for sale, or the sale or supply, in bulk, of veterinary drugs.

It must be noted that this is a much more restricted provision than the agricultural requisites of PML drugs.

i) The drug must be sold for incorporation in animal feeding stuffs.
ii) The sale must be to a person whom the seller knows or has reasonable cause to believe to be a person carrying on a business wholly or mainly comprising the manufacture of animal feeding stuffs for sale. This requirement does not preclude the sale or supply of certain veterinary drugs listed in Schedule 1, parts A and B, to farmers for "home-mixing".
iii) No sale by self service methods.
iv) A record must be kept giving the date of sale, name, quantity, form and strength, and the name and address of the purchaser. Invoices or orders, or copies thereof, will suffice. Records must be kept for two years.
v) An unqualified person must register with the Royal Pharmaceutical Society (in Northern Ireland, the Department of Agriculture) and renew each year in case of change. The details of _every_ premises where veterinary drugs will be sold must be given.

Detailed conditions appertaining to the sale and incorporation of medicinal products in feed are given in Chapter 12.

Codes of practice

The Royal College of Veterinary Surgeons and the Royal Pharmaceutical Society have professional codes of conduct for their members which supplement regulations and must be observed to maintain professional registration. The Royal Pharmaceutical Society's Practice Committee and its Agricultural and Veterinary Committee give advice to the members of the Society. Animal health distributors obtain advice from Animal Health Distributors Association (AHDA) and saddlers from the British Equestrian Trade Association (BETA).

Mention was made earlier of the Code of Practice for merchants. This has been prepared by representatives from manufacturers' and distributors' trade associations, the National Farmers Union, the veterinary associations and Royal Pharmaceutical Society together with the Ministry of Agriculture, Fisheries and Food. Applicants for registration as an animal health distributor undertake to observe this, which contains many procedures additional to the regulations. Although not law, it has a quasi-legal effect, can affect registration and in the case of a prosecution under the regulations, non-observance would be taken into account. The reference is Ministry of Agriculture Booklet PB 0769 1991 for merchants and PB 0768 for saddlers, obtainable from the Ministry or the relevant trade association and every animal health distributor and saddler should have a copy.

The promotion and advertising of animal medicines by manufacturers is controlled by the "Code of Practice for the Promotion of Animal Medicines", administered by NOAH. Copies of the Code are available free of charge from The Secretary, Code of Practice, 3 Crossfield Chambers, Gladbeck Way, Enfield EN2 7HF.

Notes
1. The Medicines (Veterinary Drugs)(Prescription Only) Order 1991 SI No 1392
2. The Medicines (Veterinary Drugs)(Pharmacy and Merchants' List) Order 1992 SI No 33. The Medicines (Pharmacy and General Sale Exemption) Order 1977 SI No 2135 Products exempted from licensing requirements prepared for retail sale in a registered pharmacy also fall into this category
3. The Medicines (Exemptions from Restrictions on the Retail Sale or Supply of Veterinary Drugs) Order 1984, as amended
4. The Medicines (Veterinary Drugs) (General Sale List) Order 1994 SI No 768

Chapter 2

Controlled Drugs
(The Misuse of Drugs Act 1971)

Dr W Derek Tavernor

The term "controlled drugs" is used to describe those compounds listed in Schedule 2 to the Misuse of Drugs Act 1971. The Act restricts the production, supply and possession of controlled drugs and provides for the issue of licences covering import and export.

The Misuse of Drugs Act 1971 established an Advisory Council on the Misuse of Drugs whose function is to review the misuse of drugs and advise Ministers on these matters. The Act, apart from giving the Home Secretary the power to make regulations to prevent the misuse of controlled drugs enables him tto take action against veterinarians who prescribe controlled drugs in an irresponsible manner. It also allows a police officer or other authorised person to enter premises used for production or supply for the purposes of inspecting books and documents relating to, and stocks of, such drugs.

The Misuse of Drugs Regulations 1985 enable certain persons, including veterinarians, to use or cause to be used, controlled drugs in the practice of their profession. Selective controls are applied to groups of drugs which are defined in Schedules to the Regulations. There are five schedules of which Schedules 2 and 3 are, in practical terms, the most important.

Schedule 1 has no real application to veterinary practice. This schedule lists the most strictly controlled drugs of all, eg raw opium, coca leaf and hallucinogens which have no relevance to everyday practice, and for the possession of which a special licence is required from the Home Secretary.

Schedule 2 is the most wide-ranging of the five schedules, over a hundred drugs being specified as well as their derivatives. They include etorphine and quinalbarbitone. The list of drugs in Schedule 2 is not as formidable as it looks: relatively few are in medical or veterinary use and very few indeed are in common use. Many drugs in this and the other schedules are included to meet the obligations of the United Nations Single Convention on Narcotic Drugs, 1961 or of the United Nations Convention on Psychotropic Substances, 1971.

Schedule 3 is the most significant, in veterinary terms. It includes barbiturates such as butobarbitone, pentobarbitone and phenobarbitone (within the generic description "5, 5 - disubstituted barbituric acids").
Schedule 4 consists mainly of benzodiazepine drugs.

Schedule 5 needs to be considered in conjunction with Schedule 2. It comprises preparations of certain controlled drugs combined with other substances in such small amounts or in such ways that they are not liable to cause harm if misused.

Possession, supply and production

A veterinary surgeon acting in his professional capacity has authority to produce, possess and supply drugs specified in Schedules 2, 3, 4 and 5. He may administer or direct any other person to adminster such drugs to animals in their care. Similarly a pharmacist may produce, possess and supply against a veterinarian's prescription controlled drugs listed in Schedules 2, 3, 4 and 5. An animal owner may possess a drug specified in these schedules if it has been supplied on a prescription from his veterinary surgeon. It is unlawful for a person to make a false statement for the purpose of obtaining a controlled drug.

(It should be noted that the Regulations empower the Home Secretary to issue a licence to approved persons, other than veterinary surgeons, to possess controlled drugs for the purpose of anaesthetising or immobilising animals).

Prescriptions

A prescription containing a controlled drug issued by a veterinary surgeon must be in ink (or otherwise indelible) and must be signed by him with his usual signature and dated by him. The prescription must have written on it the words 'for animal treatment only'.

To minimise the possibility of forging or alteration of the prescription the following details must be in the veterinary surgeon's own handwriting:

a) The name and address of the owner of the animal.
b) The dose to be given, the form eg tablets or capsules, and, where appropriate, the strength of the preparation.
c) Either the total quantity of the preparation containing the drug, or the number of dosage units to be supplied, must be written in both words and figures.
d) In the case of a prescription to be dispensed by instalments, the number of instalments and intervals to be observed when dispensing must be specified along with the amount of drug in the instalment, and the total amount of drug to be dispensed.

No prescription for a drug can be dispensed:

a) unless it complies with the above provisions;
b) unless the address of the prescriber is one in the United Kingdom,
c) unless the dispenser is acquainted with the signature of the prescriber or has no reason to suppose that it is not genuine,
d) before the date given in the prescription, or
e) later than 13 weeks after the date given in the prescription.

Registers

Registers must be kept by veterinarians for recording all transactions in respect of drugs specified in Schedules 1 and 2. The layout of registers is given in Schedule 6 of the Misuse of Drugs Regulations 1985 and is as shown.

Form of a Register

Part 1
Entries to be made in case of obtaining supply

Date on which supply received	Name Address of person or firm from whom obtained	Amount obtained	Form in which obtained

Part II
Entries to be made in case of supply

Date on which the transaction was effected	Name Address of person or firm supplied	Particulars as to licence or authority of person or firm supplied to be in possession	Amount supplied	Form in which supplied

A register must be bound (not a loose leaf book) but need not be printed. Any bound book is sufficient if appropriately ruled with the columns appropriately headed. Printed registers can however be purchased from some publishers. Entries in the register must be made in chronological order giving particulars of every quantity of a drug specified in Schedule 1 or 2 obtained, and of every quntity of drug supplied, whether by way of administration or otherwise. *(It is not necessary for a veterinary surgeon to enter drugs supplied to a patient on prescription and dispensed by a pharmacists).*

A separate register, or part of a register, must be used for each class of drugs. A class is any of the drugs specified in paragrahps 1 and 3 of Schedule 1 and paragraphs 1, 3 and 6 of Schedule 2, together with its salts and stereoisomers, and also includes preparations containing these drugs. If a preparation contains more than one class of drug subject to record-keeping requirements, an entry must be made on each page of the register, assigned to the different classes of drugs involved. (As far as the majority of veterinary surgeons are concerned this would only apply to Schedule 2, paragraphs 1 and 6.) Entries must be made on the day on which drugs are obtained or supplied, or if this is not practicable on the next day. No entry may be cancelled, obliterated, or altered. Any correction must be by marginal note, or footnote, giving the date on which the correction is made. All entries and corrections must be in ink or otherwise indelible.

A register must not be used for any purpose other than that described in the regulations, and must be produced on the demand of the Secretary of State or a person authorised in writing by him, along with any stock of drugs that are held.

A separate register must be kept for each set of premises where a stock of drugs is held. Each register must relate only to drugs obtained at, or supplied from, those premises, and must be kept on the premises to which it relates. Registers must be retained for two years from the date of the last entry.

Destruction of controlled drugs

No person required to keep a register of transactions for controlled drugs may destroy a controlled drug except in the presence of a person authorised by the Secretary of State. A record must be made of the date of destruction and the quantity destroyed which must be signed by the authorised person.

The Misuse of Drugs (Safe Custody) Regulations 1973 require that all controlled drugs from Schedule 1 and 2 (with the exception of quinalbarbitone) and the Schedule 3 drugs diethylproprion and buprenorphine must be kept in a locked receptacle which can only be opened by the veterinary surgeon or somebody authorised by him to open it (see Chapter 5).

It is most important that all veterinary surgeons and pharmacists fully understand their obligations and responsibilities in the supply, storage and recording of all transactions relating to controlled drugs.

Further information and advice relating to controlled drugs may be obtained from Drugs Branch, Home Office, Queen Anne's Gate, London SW1H 9AT.

MISUSE OF DRUGS RELATIONS 1985 (AS AMENDED)

SCHEDULE 1

CONTROLLED DRUGS SUBJECT TO THE REQUIREMENTS OF REGULATIONS 14, 15, 16, 18, 19, 20, 23, 25 AND 26

1. The following substances and products, namely:-

   (a) Bufotenine
   Cannabinol
   Cannabinol derivatives (not being dronabinol or its stereoisomers)
   Cannabis and cannabis resin
   Cathinone
   Coca leaf
   Concentrate of poppy-straw
   Eticyclidine
   Lysergamide
   Lysergide and other N-alkyl derivaties of lysergamide
   Mescaline
   Psilocin
   Raw opium
   Rolicyclidine
   Tenocyclidine
   4-Bromo-2, 5-dimethoxy-&-methylphenethylamine
   N, N-Diethyltryptamine
   N, N-Dimethyltryptamine
   2, 5-Dimethoxy-*L*, 4-dimethylphenethylamine
   N Hydroxy
   4-Methyl

   (b) any compound (not being a compound for the time being specified in sub-paragraph (a) above) structually derived from tryptamine or from a ring-hydroxy tryptamine by substitution at the nitrogen atom of the sidechain with one or more alkyl substituents but no other substituent;

   (c) any compound (not being methoxyphenamine or a compound for the time being specified in sub-paragraph (a) above) structually derived from phenethylamine, an N-alkylphenethylamine, *a*-methylphenethylamine, or an N-alkyl-*a*-ethylphenethylamine by substitution in the ring to any extent with alkyl, alkoxy, alkylenedioxy or halide substituents, whether or not further substituted in the ring by one or more other univalent substituents;

(d) any compound (not being a compound for the time being specified in Schedule 2) structually derived from fentanyl by modification in any of the following ways, that is to say,

   (i)   by replacements of the phenyl portion of the phenethyl group by any heteromonocycle whether or not further substituted in the heterocycle;
   (ii)   by substitution in the phenethyl group with alkyl, alkenyl, alkoxy, hydroxy, halogeno, haloalkyl, amino or nitro groups;
   (iii)   by substitution in the piperidine ring with alkyl or alkenyl groups;
   (iv)   by substitution in the aniline ring with alkyl, alkoxy, alkyl-enedioxy, halogeno or haloalkyl groups;
   (v)   by substitution at the 4-position of the piperidine ring with any alkoxycarbonyl or alkoxyalkyl or acyloxy group;
   (vi)   by replacement of the N-propionyl group by another acyl group;

(e) any compound (not being a compound for the time being specified in Schedule 2) structurally derived from pethidine by modification in any of the following ways, that is to say,

   (i)   by replacement of the 1-methyl group by an acyl, alkyl whether or not unsaturated, benzyl or phenethyl group, whether or not further substituted.
   (iii)   by substitution in the piperidine ring with alkyl or alkenyl groups or with a propano bridge, whether or not further substituted;
   (iii)   by substitution in the 4-phenyl ring with alkyl, alkoxy, aryloxy, halogeno or haloalkyl groups;
   (iv)   by replacement of the 4-ethoxycarbonyl by any other alkoxycarbonyl or any alkoxyalkyl or acyloxy group;
   (v)   by formation of an N-oxide or of a quaternary base.

2. Any stereoisomeric form of a substance specified in paragraph 1.

3. Any ester or ether of a substance specified in paragraph 1 or 2.

4. Any salt of a substance specified in any of paragraphs 1 to 3.

5. Any preparation or other product containing a substance or product specified in any of paragraphs 1 to 4, not being a preparation specified in Schedule 5.

SCHEDULE 2

CONTROLLED DRUGS SUBJECT TO THE REQUIREMENTS OF REGULATIONS 14, 15, 16, 18. 19, 20, 21, 23, 25 and 26

1. The following substances and products, namely:-

Acetorphine
Alfentanil
Allylprodine
Alphacetylmethadol
Alphameprodine
Alphamethadol
Alphaprodine
Anileridine
Benzethidine
Benzylmorphine
    (3-benzylmorphine)
Betacetylmethadol
Betaprodine
Bezitramide
Carfentanil
Clonitazene
Cocaine
Desomorphine
Dextromoramide
Diamorphine
Diampromide
Diethylthiambutene
Difenoxin
Dihydrocodeinone
    O-carboxymethyloxime
Dihydromorphine
Dimenoxadole
Dimepheptanol
Dimethylthiambutene
Dioxaphetyl butyrate
Diphenoxylate
Dipipanone
Dronabinol
Drotebanol

Ecgonine, and any derivative
    of ecgonine which is convertible
    to ecogonine or to cocaine
Ethylmethylthiambutene
Etonitazene
Etorphine
Etoxeridine
Fentanyl
Furethidine
Hydrocodone
Hydromorphinol
Hydromorphone
Hydroxypethidine
Isomethadone
Ketobemidone
Levomethorphan
Levomoramide
Levophenacylmorphan
Levorphanol
Lofentanil
Medicinal opium
Metazocine
Methadone
Methadyl acetate
Methyldesorphine
Methyldihydromorphine
    (6-methyldihydromorphine)
Metopan
Morpheridine
Morphine
Morphine methobromide,
    morphine N-oxide and other
    pentavalent nitrogen morphine
    derivatives

Myrophine
Nicomorphine
Noracymethadol
Norlevorphanol
Normethadone
Normorphine
Norpipanone
Oxycodone
Oxymorephone
Pethidine
Phenadoxone
Phenampromide
Phenazocine
Phencyclidine
Phenomorphan
Phenoperidine
Piminodine
Piritramide
Proheptazine
Properidine

Racemethorphan
Racemoramide
Racemorphan
Sufentanil
Thebacon
Thebaine
Tilidate
Trimeperidine
4-Cyano-2-dimethylamino-4, 4-diphenylbutane
4-Cyano-1-methyl-4-phenylpiperidine
1-Methyl-4-phenylpiperidine-4-carboxylic acid
2-Methyl-3-morpholino-1, 1-diphenylpropanecarboxylic acid
4-Phenylpiperidine-4-carboxylic acid ethyl ester

2. Any stereoisomeric form of a substance specified in paragraph 1 not being dextromethorphan or dextrorphan.

3. Any ester or ether of a substance specified in paragraph 1 or 2, not being a substance specified in paragraph 6.

4. Any salt of a substance specified in any of paragraphs 1 to 3.

5. Any preparation or other product containing a substance or product specified in any of paragraphs 1 to 4, not being a preparation specified in Schedule 5.

6. The following substances and products, namely:-

Acetyldihydrocodeine
Amphetamine
Codeine
Dextropropoxypehene
Dhydrocodeine
Ethylmorphine (3-ethylmorphine)
Fenethylline
Glutethimide
Lefetamine

Mecloqualone
Methaqualone
Methylamphetamine
Methylphenidate
Nicocodine
Nicodicodine (6-nicotinoyldihydrocodeine)
Norcodeine
Phenmetrazine

Pholcodine
Propiram
Quinalbarbitone

7. Any stereoisomeric form of a substance specified in paragraph 6.

8. Any salt of a substances specified in paragraph 6 or 7.

9. Any preparation or other product containing a substance or product specified in any of paragraphs 6 to 8, not being a preparation specified in Schedule 5.

SCHEDULE 3

CONTROLLED DRUGS SUBJECT TO THE REQUIREMENTS OF REGULATIONS 14, 15, 16, 18, 22, 23, 24, 25 and 26

1. The following substances, namely:

   (a) Benzphetamine
   Buprenorphine
   Cathine
   Chlorphentermine
   Diethylpropion
   Ethchlorvynol
   Ethinamate
   Mazindol
   Mephentermine
   Meprobamate
   Methylphenobarbitone
   Methyprylone
   Pentazocine
   Phendimetrazine
   Phentermine
   Pipradrol

   (b) any 5,5 disubstituted barbituric acid, not being quinalbarbitone.

2. Any stereoisomeric form of a substance specified in paragraph 1, not being phenylpropanolamine.

3. Any salt of a substance specified in paragraph 1 or 2.

4. Any preparation or other product containing a substance specified in any of paragraphs 1 to 3, not being a preparation specified in Schedule 5.

SCHEDULE 4

CONTROLLED DRUGS EXCEPTED FROM THE PROHIBITION ON IMPORTATION, EXPORTATION AND, WHEN IN THE FORM OF A MEDICINAL PRODUCT, POSSESSION AND SUBJECT TO THE REQUIREMENTS OF REGULATIONS 22, 23, 25 and 26.

1. The following substances and products, namely:

Alprazolam	Loprazolam
Bromazepam	Lorazepam
Camazepam	Lormetazepam
Chlordiazepoxide	Medazepam
Clobazam	Mefenorex
Clonazepic acid	Midazolam
Clotiazepam	Nimetazepam
Cloxazolam	Nitrazepam
Delorazepam	Nordazepam
Diazepam	Oxazepam
Estazolam	Oxazolam
Ethyl loflazepate	Pemoline
Fencamfamin	Pinazepam
Fenproporex	Prazepam
Fludiazepam	Propylhexedrine
Flunitrazepam	Pyrovalerone
Flurazepam	Temazepam
Halazepam	Tetrazepam
Haloxazolam	Triazolam
Ketazolam	N-Ethylamphetamine

2. Any stereoisomeric form of a substance specified in paragraph 1.

3. Any salt of a substance specified in paragraph 1 or 2.

4. Any preparation or other product containing a substance or product specified in any of paragraphs 1 to 3, not being a preparation specified in Schedule 5.

SCHEDULE 5

CONTROLLED DRUGS EXCEPTED FROM THE PROHIBITION ON IMPORTATION, EXPORTATION AND POSSESSION AND SUBJECT TO THE REQUIREMENTS OF REGULATIONS 24 and 25.

1. (i) Any preparation of one or more of the substances to which this paragraph applied, not being a preparation designed for administration by injection, when compounded with one or more other active or inert ingredients and containing a total of not more than 100 milligrammes of the substances or substances (calculated as base) per dosage unit or with a total concentration of not more than 2.5 per cent (calculated as base) in undivided preparations.
   (ii) The substances to which this paragraph applies are acetyldihydrocodeine, codeine, dihydrocodeine, ethylmorphine, nicocodine, nicodicodine (6-nicotinoyldihydrocodeine), norcodeine, pholcodine and their respective salts.

2. Any preparation of cocaine containing not more than 0.1 per cent of cocaine calculated as cocaine base, being a preparation compounded with one or more other active or inert ingredients in such a way that the cocaine cannot be recovered by readily applicable means or in a yield which would constitute a risk to health.

3. Any preparation of medicinal opium or of morphine containing (in either case) not more than 0.2 per cent of morphine calculated as anhydrous morphine base, being a preparation compounded with one or more other active or inert ingredients in such a way that the opium or, as the case may be, the morphine cannot be recovered by readily applicable means or in a yield which would constitute a risk to health.

4. Any preparation of dextropropoxyphene, being a preparation designed for oral administration, containing not more than 135 milligrammes of dextropropoxyphene (calculated as base) per dosage unit or with a total concentration of not more than 2.5 per cent (calculated as base) in undivided preparations.

5. Any preparation of difenoxin containing, per dosage unit, not more than 0.5 milligrammes of difenoxin and a quantity of atropine sulphate equivalent to at least 5 per cent of the dose of difenoxin.

6. Any preparation of diphenoxylate containing per dosage unit, not more than 2.5 milligrammes of difenoxin and a quantity of atropine sulphate equivalent to at least 5 per cent of the dose of difenoxin.

7. Any preparation of propiram containing, per dosage unit, not more than 100 milligrammes of propiram calculated as base and compounded with at least the same amount (by weight) of methylcellulose.

8. Any powder of ipecacuanha and opium comprising:

   10 per cent opium, in powder
   10 per cent ipecacuanha root, in powder, well mixed with 80 per cent of any other powdered ingredient containing no controlled drug.

9. Any mixture containing one or more of the preparations specified in paragraphs 1 to 8, being a mixture of which none of the other ingredients is a controlled drug. *

   NB: The government propose to bring anabolic steroids and a number of other anabolic/androgenic substances under the controls of the Misuse of Drugs legislation.

Chapter 3

Health & Safety at Work, etc Act 1974

R E Ablett revised by Cameron N Downie

The Health and Safety at Work, etc Act 1974 is an enabling Act which draws together all previous legislation and allows for new regulations to be made. It extends previous legislation to all work places[1]. A breach of statutory duty under the Act can give rise to criminal liability for which both the organisation and its senior employees can be held responsible[2]. The purpose of the Act is described in the introduction as follows:

An act to make further provision for securing the health, safety and welfare of persons at work, for protecting others against risks to health or safety in connection with the activities of persons at work, for controlling the keeping and use and preventing the unlawful acquisition, possession and use of dangerous substances, and for controlling certain emissions into the atmosphere.

A detailed account of the Health and Safety at Work, etc Act is beyond the scope of this publication. Further information can be obtained from some of the references given at the end of the chapter.

General duties
The intention of the Act is clearly to secure the health and safety not only of those who work but also for others against hazards arising out of work. For those who employ, who are employed or who are self employed, this piece of legislation relates to WORK and whichever aspect of the Act is under examination it must be associated with work[3].

There is a general duty for employers to ensure, as far as is reasonably practicable, the health, safety and welfare of his employees, particularly in the maintenance of plant and systems of work in avoiding hazards connected with the use, handling, storage and transport of articles and substances, and providing information, instruction, training, supervision, and overall to provide a safe working environment. Employers of more than four employees are required, under the Act, to provide a written safety policy which must be brought to the notice of all employees. This safety policy should help employers decide on priorities, detail health and safety objectives and outline the organization that exists for ensuring they are met. It should also set out how the policy is to be implemented.

There is a similar general duty for employers and self-employed to ensure, so far as is reasonably practicable, the safety of others who may be affected by their work.

On the other hand, an employee must himself take reasonable care for the health and safety of himself and others, and must co-operate so far as it necessary with his employer regarding any duty imposed on his employer. The motto 'Safety is Everyone's Business' conveys the spirit aptly.

General duties of manufacturers, etc.
The Act specifically defines the duties of persons who manufacture articles and substances for use at work. They must arrange for necessary tests to be performed that will eliminate or minimize any risk when the product is properly used. The Act does not require any person to repeat any testing if such testing can reasonably be expected to be reliable.

In addition to the above, manufacturers, importers and suppliers must take necessary steps to supply adequate information about the use for which the substance or article is intended, and for which it has been tested to ensure that it is safe and without risk to health when properly used. This part of the Act [4] is important to those who, for example, manufacture, supply, import or dispense animal medicines.

The primary responsibility for the safety of animal medicines rests (in so far as they affect the workforce and others) with the manufacturer or importer and it is his duty to package, test and label correctly. This responsibility will however shift to the supplier if the supplier in any way alters the packaging, changes the product, or alters the labelling in any material way. For example, a corrosive substance correctly labelled would become a risk to safety if it was to be refilled into unsuitable containers. Responsibility passes to the person undertaking the refilling. Similarly, persons 'breaking bulk' or dispensing dangerous substances would become responsible for giving adequate warning of the possible dangers that may exist to persons using that substance at work. The person undertaking the refilling must also take necessary precautions for the safety of persons in his employment who handle the compound.

Enforcement
Provision is made for two corporate bodies under the Health and Safety at Work, etc Act 1974. The Health and Safety Commission (consisting of a Chairman and up to nine members) is a policy making body which also directs the work of the Health and Safety Executive (HSE prepare legislation on behalf of the Commission. It is then sent to the Secretary of State who

lays it before Parliament before it becomes law. The HSE are also responsible for organizing the day to day administration of health and safety legislation). The Health and Safety Executive inspector has wide powers; he may at any reasonable time enter premises and make such examinations and investigate as necessary for the purpose of satisfying himself as to the necessary standards of safety. If he feels a situation may be dangerous then he may enter at any time. If danger appear to exist, these powers are wide enough to allow him to, for example, take measurements, photographs, samples or even take into possession or dismantle so to prevent further use. He may merely serve 'an improvement notice' or a 'prohibition notice' preventing a specific operation or process which can sometimes effectively close the premises until it is rectified. On the other hand inspectors spend most of their time in an advisory capacity and it is unlikely that prohibition or improvement notices are served in the first instance. Often inspectors under the Health and Safety at Work, etc Act work closely with fire prevention officers, particularly where flammable materials are stored.

The inspectors look for dangerous working conditions associated with the safety of structures, machines and operations, for example, and are alert to the presence of any acute or toxic hazard arising from chemical or electrical sources, in addition to the risk of fire. They are also concerned with safety precautions and how these are implemented. Particular reference might be made to unsatisfactory storage, bad racking and shelving, trailing wires and sharp projections, heating and ventilation where dangerous chemicals, gases and powders are handled. Safe access and exits, the causes of accidents, dust control and methods of working are important. The areas mentioned demonstrate the wide implications of the Act, and are not intended as a checklist.

Since the Act was passed it has become obvious that one of the major risks to health in veterinary practice is the use of X-ray machines. Not only must the machine itself be safe and regularly serviced, but satisfactory protection must be available to the veterinary surgeon's staff in the form of clothing, education, and warning. The siting of the machine is very important for the protection of employees, clients and visitors to the premises. There is no doubt that practices will be visited with this particular point in mind. The Guidance Notes for the Protection of Persons against Ionising Radiations arising from Veterinary Use is a useful publication for reference. Also less obvious risks should not be forgotten such as the risk of infection from animals and the risk of inadvertent injection.

Offences
Persons guilty of offences under certain parts of the Act will be liable on summary conviction to a fine not exceeding £2,000. Under other parts of the penalty may be a fine on summary conviction of a sum not exceeding £2,000 but on conviction on indictment, the penalty may be an unlimited fine or imprisonment for a term not exceeding 2 years for certain offences, or both. In any proceedings for an offence under any of the relevant provisions of the Act it shall be for the accused to prove that it was not practicable or not reasonably practicable to do more than what was in fact done to satisfy the duty or requirement, or that there was no better practicable means than was in fact used to satisfy the duty or requirement.

The Act also lays down provisions for appeal against notices served, or refusal to grant necessary licences where these are required.

It is interesting to note that special provisions relate to agriculture. The Minister of Agriculture, Fisheries and Food has a power and, indeed a duty, to make special health and safety regulations for relevant agricultural purposes. These will be made from time to time jointly with the Secretary of State for Employment. There are other occasions when the Secretary of State for Employment makes legislation on his own. In this respect the Agriculture Minister works with the Secretary of State on regulations applying to Great Britain, whereas in respect to other parts of the Act, the 'Commission' and the 'Executive' work with the Secretary of State alone.

Management of Health & Safety at Work Regulations 1992 (MHSWR)
The Health and Safety at Work, etc Act 1974 (HSAW) set out the basic framework for the successful management of health and safety at work. This framework has been much extended by the introduction of the Management of Health and Safety at Work Regulations 1992 (MHSWR). Regulation 4 of MHSWR states that the fundamental principles of successful management of health and safety at work involve:

.... the effective planning, organisation, control, monitoring and review of the preventative and protective measures.
This health and safety management system of planning, organisation, control and monitoring forms the basis of the legal requirements and should therefore be the starting point for a successful health and safety plan. Such a plan is unlikely to succeed without the commitment of senior managers and acceptance of health and safety responsibilities by employees.

In order to fulfil obligations under MHSWR, the employer will need to establish procedures for a wide range of health and safety at work topics, including as a minimum:-

1. keeping up to date with health & safety legislation
2. arrangements for undertaking risk assessments
3. safety training
4. safety communications
5. safety committees and safety representatives
6. disciplinary procedures
7. records and registers
8. fire safety standards
9. first aid at work
10. accident procedures
11. medical and health surveillance requirements
12. control of contractors on site
13. visits by employees to other locations
14. enforcing authority visits
15. monitoring health and safety at work

Risk Assessments

The MHSWR require suitable and sufficient assessments of the risks to health and safety arising from work activities. The wide range of risk assessments which must be undertaken will all be consolidated in the health and safety policy statement. Persons responsible for the management of health and safety must ensure that suitable and sufficient risk assessments are undertaken to a suitable standard, within an acceptable timescale and are recorded in a consistent and satisfactory format. The responsibilities related to undertaking and recording risk assessment should be detailed in the responsibilities section of the health and safety policy.

Control of Substances Hazardous to Health ('COSHH') Regulations 1994 (see also Chapter 4)

The Regulations relate to work involving substances which are defined as being hazardous to health. The Regulations require that employers do not carry out any work involving substances hazardous to health unless a suitable and sufficient assessment has been made of the risks to health created by the work and the measures necessary to control exposure to substances hazardous to health. The employer must ensure that such exposure is prevented or controlled. Control measures must be maintained, examined, tested and properly used. In certain circumstances monitoring of exposure to substances hazardous to health and health surveillance should be carried out. Employers must provide their employees with such information, instruction and training to ensure that they know the risks to health created by exposure to substances hazardous to health and the precautions which must be taken.

Under the COSHH regulations the manufacturers of animal medicines now provide product safety data sheets to a format agreed with HSE to aid customer assessment of risk to their employees. The British Veterinary Association Guide to the initial assessment in veterinary practices is available from the British Veterinary Association, 7 Mansfield Street, London W1M OAT.

Other Relevant Legislation
Specific requirements on health, safety and welfare in the workplace are laid down in the following Acts and Regulations

1. the Factories Act 1961;
2. the Office Shops and Railway Premises Act 1963;
3. the Electricity at Work Regulations 1989;
4. the Control of Substances Hazardous to Health Regulations 1994
5. the Noise at Work Regulations 1989;
6. the Protection of Eye Regulations 1974;
7. the Pressure Systems and Transportable Gas Containers Regulations 1989;
8. the Highly Flammable Liquids and Liquified Petroleum Gases Regulations 1972;
9. the Reporting of Injuries on Dangerous Occurrences Regulations 1977;
10. the Health & Safety (First Aid) Regulations 1981;
11. the Safety Representatives and Safety Committees Regulations 1977;
12. the Fire Precautions Act 1971;
13. the Food and Environmental Protection Act 1985;
14. the Control of Pesticides Regulations 1986;
15. the Safety Signs Regulations 1980;
16. the Management of Health and Safety at Work Regulations 1992;
17. the Workplace (Health, Safety and Welfare) Regulations 1992;
18. the Personal Protective Equipment at Work Regulations 1992;
19. the Provision and Use of Work Equipment Regulations 1992;
20. the Health and Safety (Display Screen Equipment) Regulations 1992;
21. the Manual Handling Regulations 1992;
22. the Chemical (Hazard Information and Packaging for Supply) Regulations 1994;
23. the Carriage of Dangerous Goods by Road and Rail (Classification, Packaging and Labelling) Regulations 1994.

Notes

[1] Many of the original statutes and regulations that relate to health and safety still remain in force. Lists of relevant statutory provision are contained in the appendices of a leaflet by the Health and Safety Commission (HSC 2). This and other leaflets in the same series can be obtained from branches of HMSO.

[2] Section 37 (1) Health and Safety at Work, etc Act 1974.

[3] It should be emphasised that the Act covers all risks to health and safety of workers arising out of the manufacture, formulation, storage, packaging, transport, dispensing and administration of animal medicines, feedstuffs, etc. These include structural defects, fire, dangerous machinery, falls, falling objects, electrical hazards, etc. as well as the more specific acute or chronic toxic hazards that may pertain to the particular materials being considered, and which will necessitate appropriate design of plant and equipment together with engineering methods (eg local exhaust ventilation) to control the emission of dust or fumes to the workplace, supplemented by personal protective measures against contact or inhalation.

[4] Section 6 Health and Safety at Work, etc. Act 1974.

Further Reading

Health and Safety Commission Leaflets:
HSC 2 - The Act outline
HSC3 - Advice to employers
HSC 4 - Advice to self-employed
HSC 5 - Advice to employees
HSC 6 - Notes on employers' policy statements for Health & Safety
HSC 8 - Safety Committees
Codes of Practice (COP):
COP 1 - Safety representatives and safety committees
ACOP - Control of Substances Hazardous to Health ISBN 0-71761-0819-0
Health and Safety Guidance (HS(G)
HS(G)65 - Successful health and safety management
Legal Series (L):
L1 - A guide to the HSW Act
L21 - Management of Health and Safety at Work Regulations 1992
Industry Guidance (IND):
IND(G)132(L) - Five steps to successful health and safety management
IND(G)163(L) - Five steps to risk assessment
HSE - Introducing COSHH
HSE - Introducing Assessment
HSE - Hazard & Risk Explained
HSE - COSHH Assessments HMSO ISBN 011 885 4704
HMSO - Step by Step Guide to COSHH assessment ISBN - 0-11-886379-7
HMSO - Farm Wise Guide to Health & Safety ISBN - 0-11-882107-5
HMSO - Essential of Health & Safety at Work ISBN - 0-11-885445-3
HMSO - Veterinary Medicines (COSHH) - Safe Use - ISBN - 0-11-886361-4

Chapter 4

Implementation of COSHH Legislation on Industry

Cameron N Downie

Introduction

Suppliers and users of animal medicines like any other employer have to discharge their duties under the Health and Safety at Work, etc Act 1974 (HSWA) to ensure the health, safety and welfare of employees. In relation to exposure to hazardous substances, the major legislation under HSWA is the Control of Substance Hazardous to Health Regulations 1994 (COSHH). These regulations represent a consensus regarding good practice in the area of prevention and control of exposure to hazardous substances. This chapter gives a brief overview of the regulations and guidance on particular aspects of implementation.

Comprehensive guidance is provided in the Approved Codes of Practice: Control of Substances Hazardous to Health (the General ACOP); and the Control of Carcinogenic Substances (the Carcinogens ACOP) and the Control of Biological Agents (the Biological Agents ACOP) published in one document. A list of other useful documents is at the back of the chapter.

General COSHH requirements

The basic principles of occupational hygiene underlie the COSHH regulations. The regulations aim to protect workers and others from adverse effects of exposure to substances hazardous to health. This is achieved by requiring employers to:-

1. Assess the risk to health arising from work involving exposure to substances hazardous to health and identify the required precaution (Regulation 6).

2. Introduce appropriate measures to prevent or adequately control the risk (Regulation 7).

3. Ensure that control measures are used and that equipment is properly maintained and procedures observed (Regulations 8 & 9).

4. Where necessary, monitor the exposure of the workers and carry out an appropriate form of surveillance of their health (Regulations 10 & 11).

5. Inform, instruct and train employees about the risks and the precautions that need to be taken (Regulation 12).

Duties and responsibilties

Employers have a range of duties to their employees. These duties also apply to other persons, so far as is reasonable practicable, who may be affected by the work. Employees have a duty to make full and proper use of control measures and personal protective equipment (Regulation 8(2)) and also, to present himself for health surveillance. Effective control of health risks depends on co-operation and co-ordination of activities. This is particularly important where a number of employees and their employers may be involved in an operation. The guiding principle is that whoever is in control of an operation must ensure that adequate arrangements are in place.

What is a substance hazardous to health?

Substances that are considered hazardous to health under the Control of Substances Hazardous to Health Regulations 1994 include:

* substances classified and labelled as very toxic, toxic, harmful, irritant or corrosive under the Chemicals (Hazard Information and Packaging for supply) Regulations 1994;

* substances specified in Schedule 1 of the COSHH Regulations (which lists substances assigned maximum exposure limits - MELs) or for which the Health and Safety Executive has an approved occupational exposure standard (OES) - see current edition of HSE publication EH40);

* a biological agent - harmful micro-organisms, dusts of any kind, when present at a substantial concentration in air;

* any substance that creates a hazard to health of any person that is comparable with the hazards created by substances mentioned above+

+ Note, this would include certain veterinary medicines and other animal health products. Not all veterinary medicines are considered hazardous in their final packed form. Certain products may have a "potentially" adverse effect on health if exposure (via inhalation, ingestion, inoculation or skin contact) were to occur. Suppliers and manufacturers have a duty under Section 6 of the Health and Safety at Work, etc Act 1974 to provide "suitable and sufficient" information on product hazards, if they exist. For "hazardous" products, this information is normally supplied by the manufacturer in the form of a material safety data sheet, or on the label or product information/

data sheet or package insert. It is not possible to comply with the requirement of the COSHH regulations without first correctly identifying those substances, preparations or products that are considered hazardous. The supplier or manufacturers should be contacted if there is any uncertainty over the hazards posed by any product.

Risk Assessment

Risk assessment is a qualitative or quantitative evaluation of the likelihood that a particular hazard will cause harm. It takes into account all the factors that effect the likelihood of ill health; and reaches conclusions about the need to improve measures to eliminate or reduce the risk to an acceptable level. The assessment is no more than a systematic examination of what substances could cause harm so that you can decide whether or not enough precautions have been taken.

A formal assessment system is proof that a particular organization has recognized the health hazards and has implemented, or is about to do so, steps to eliminate or minimize their incidence. The purpose of an assessment is to identify the measures necessary to prevent or control exposure to substances hazardous to health arising from any work.

The assessment should identify:-

* the risks posed to the health of the workforce;
* the steps necessary to control exposure to those hazards;
* any additional action required to achieve compliance with the reglations.

The assessment will involve asking questions such as:-

1. What hazardous substances are likely to be present in the workplace?
2. How are the substances are hazardous? (Eg inhalation, inoculation, ingestion, etc)
3. What are the possible harmful effects of over exposure? (Acute, chronic health effects)
4. Where are the substances used, handled or stored?
5. Who may be exposed to them and for how long?
6. What control measures currently exist (eg protective equipment)
7. Are the control measures adequate and effective?
8. What is the likelihood of exposure, given the effectiveness of existing controls?
9. How can exposure be further eliminated, prevented or controlled?

In gathering information for the assessment, you may need to take expert advice. Merely following the suppliers' product data sheets is not necessarily sufficient for compliance purposes; HSE Guidance Notes and manufacturer's standards should also be consulted. HSE guidance will be available and many manufacturers provide information on their products. In all but the simplest cases the assessment will need to be written. Anyone who may be affected by a hazardous substance must be told about the assessment.

The likelihood of exposure to a substance hazardous to health depend upon:-

- the amount of substance being used (mgs, kgs - mls, litres)
- the nature of the compound (dust, vapour, gas, liquid aerosol)
- the potential routes of exposure (inhalation, ingestion, inoculation, skin contact/absorption)
- the duration and frequency of use (minutes, hours - daily, weekly)
- the exposing potential of the activity or operation (spraying, pouring, dispensing, injecting)

All work and work practices which may involve hazardous substances should be assessed to decide on the control measures to prevent exposure. The potential for exposure via inhalation, ingestion, inoculation, skin contact or absorption needs to be evaluated and for each activity a judgement should be made on the "adequacy" of existing precautionary and/or preventative measures. For veterinary medicines deemed hazardous, typical activities requiring assessment may include:-

- Storage of material
- Transfer of materials
- Disposal of waste materials (Eg clinical waste, sharps, medicines)
- Use:-
    - Veterinary drug - oral administration (drench, feed additives, solid dose forms)
    - Veterinary drug - topical administration (lotions, pour-on, powder dip)
    - Veterinary drug -injection administration (vaccines, antibiotics)
    - Veterinary drug - preparation (dispensing, mixing)

In addition to "normal" operations, the assessment needs to consider any maintenance and cleaning operations and foreseeable emergencies (ie accidental inoculation, accidental ingestion, splashes, spillage, etc). The assessment should be used to determine the need for additional action to reduce the likelihood of an emergency event and judge the adequacy of existing emergency procedures.

It is important to assess the risk to those who may be directly or indirectly affected by the work. Other persons may need to be taken into account (ie veterinary assistants, farm workers etc) as they could be "potentially" at risk of exposure to a substance classified as hazardous to health.

The COSHH regulations also cover biological agents that have a potential to cause infection and disease. Certain special measures are required in veterinary care facilities, laboratories and animal rooms that involve the use of biological agents, to ensure that biological agents are not transmitted to workers or outside the controlled area. Due to the nature of the work, veterinary practitioners come into contact with a variety of animals and may be directly or indirectly exposed to certain occupational zoonoses. In such cases, assessments should cover exposure to occupational zoonosis and any other biological agents present. See the HSE Biological Agents ACOP (Control of biological agents) for additional guidance.

Prevention & Control

COSHH requires exposure to be prevented or, where this is not reasonably practicable, adequately controlled. The general ACOP gives a hierarchy of preferred control measures and sets out how adequate control may be achieved and recognized. The use of personal protective equipment (PPE), including respiratory protective equipment is only acceptable as a last resort in addition to other means if these alone can not provide adequate control. The provision of control measures is not sufficient in itself, you also have to ensure that they are properly applied.

On the basis of the assessment, you have to decide which control measures are appropriate to your work situation in order to deal effectively with any hazardous substances that may be present. For existing work situations, the present control measures should be carefully reviewed, and improved, extended or replaced as necessary to be capable of achieving, and sustaining adequate control. This may mean preventing exposure by:

* removing the hazardous substance
* substituting with a safe or safer substance, or using it in a safer form.

Or where this is not reasonably practicable, controlling exposure by for example:

* introducing technical or engineering methods of controlling exposure
* selection of equipment or systems that minimize the generation or contain the hazard
* reducing exposure by following safe systems of work

* use of ventilation and partial enclosures
* reduction of numbers of employees and limit exposure periods
* provision of personal protective equipment
* provision of adequate facilities for washing, changing and storage of clothing
* prohibition of eating, drinking and smoking etc. where chemicals are handled

Exposure should be controlled so that nearly all people would not suffer any adverse health effects even if they were exposed to a substance day after day. For certain substances where the risk to health is through inhalation, Occupational Exposure Limits (OELs) have been set. (See HSE Guidance Note EH 40/49.) There are two kinds of exposure limit for substances that have been given maximum exposure limits (MELs). The level of exposure should be reduced so far as is reasonably practicable and, in any event should not exceed the MEL. For other substances with occupational exposure standards, it is sufficient to ensure the level of exposure is reduced to that standard.

Respiratory protective equipment, if used, must conform with EC standards or be of a type approved by the HSE. The guidance shows that respiratory protection requires a big back-up in training, supervision and that correct fitting is crucial.

Maintenance, examination and test of control measures

COSHH places specific obligations on employers to ensure that all control measures are kept in an efficient working order and good repair. Maintenance of control measures includes checks on extraction equipment, monitoring of exposure and checking to ensure that the rules are enforced. If control measures consist of engineering controls, they should be examined and tested at suitable intervals. For example, local exhaust ventilation equipment has to be tested at least once every 14 months and a simple record kept. Respirators and breathing apparatus also have to be examined frequently.

Information, instruction and training

The General ACOP sets out what information, instruction and training should be provided by employers. Employers need to ensure that staff are competent to apply the COSHH requirements. Employees have to be informed about the health risks and should be provided with appropriate instruction and training on the correct measures to safe guard health. Work with veterinary medicines should only be carried out by persons who have been given adequate instruction and training. The assessment procedure should be used to determine whether or not those involved appreciate the risks arising from their work and understand the precautions to be taken during normal work (storage, use, disposal, cleaning, etc) and in emergencies.

Health surveillance
Guidance on when health surveillance is necessary is provided in the General ACOP and in Health Surveillance under COSHH: guidance for employers. Employers have a duty to provide health surveillance only for their employees. The need for health surveillance should be determined as part of the COSHH assessment.

Health surveillance is required if:-

1. employees are exposed to a substance linked to a specific ill health
2. there is reasonable likelihood under the conditions of work that the ill health might occur
3. it is possible to detect indications or ill-health effect

Generally, health surveillance is only necessary when there is doubt that the exposure of the individual to a potentially hazardous substance cannot be satisfactorily controlled and in consequence the worker's health may be affected. This could involve the services of a doctor or trained nurse. It could also include trained supervisors checking employees' skin for severe dermatitis, or asking questions about breathing difficulties if the work involves substances known to cause asthma. Where heatlh surveillance is carried out, a simple health record, comprising mainly basic personnel details, should be kept.

Further action
All employers need to consider how COSHH applies to their work. Failure to comply with COSHH consitutes an offence and you may be subject to prosecution. Fines of up to £2000 can be imposed or even prison sentences. For many employers, compliance with COSHH may be simple and straightforward; for others, more substantial work may be needed on assessment and the introduction and maintenance of control measures. Your local Health and Safety Inspector will be able to offer help and advice. See under Health and Safety in your telephone directory.

Publications

The following publications give more detailed information on COSHH and its requirements:

1. Introducing Assessment, leaflet available free from HSE
2. Hazard and Risk Explained, leaflet available free from HSE
3. COSHH Assessments (a step-by-step guide to assessment) HMSO, ISBN 0 11 885470 4
4. General COSHH ACOP (Control of Substances Hazardous to Health) and Carcinogens ACOP (Control of Carcinogenic Substances) Biological agents ACOP (Control of Biological Agents) control of Substances Hazardous to Health Regulations 1994 HMSO ISBN 0-7176-0819-0
5. Guidance Note EH40/94 (and subsequent editions) Occupational Exposure Limits, HMSO, ISBN 0-11-885411 9
6. Chemicals (Hazard Information and Packaging for Supply) Regulations 1994 or CHIP 2 for short - CHIP 2 for everyone HMSO ISBN 0-71-76-0857-3
7. Veterinary Medicines. Safe use by farmers and other animal handlers 1992. ISBN 0-11-882051
8. Guide to an initial assessment in veterinary practices - British Veterinary Association, 7 Mansfield Street, London W1M 0AT.

Chapter 5

Storage, Transportation and Aspects of Safety in Veterinary Practice

J Tandy revised by Bas D W Hardy

INTRODUCTION
The Medicines Act enables the Minister to introduce legislation controlling the conditions under which medicinal products are stored and transported. No such regulations specifically applicable to a veterinary practice have been enacted but there is a general expectation that the conditions specified on the product label and data sheet will be observed.

Considerable general legislation covering many aspects of the transport, storage and handling of animal medicines is now in place including COSHH and CHIP regulations. These are addressed elsewhere in this handbook and this chapter is devoted to providing advice whereby the licensed quality, safety and efficacy of animal medicines are maintained after despatch from the manufacturer or wholesaler.

GENERAL STORAGE REQUIREMENTS
The design of veterinary premises varies considerably depending on the size and type of practice, whether they are the main premises or a branch surgery etc. Medicines are present in the designated store room, the dispensary, the consulting room, the 'point of sale' and practice motor cars and are transported between branches.

In order to maintain the licensed quality, safety and efficacy of animal medicines the following should be carefully considered.

Construction and design of premises
The building or part of the building in which medicines are stored should be of a permanent nature and should be vermin proof.

The premises should be designed, equipped and organised in a manner to ensure the safe and efficient handling of products.

An excellent design principle is to divide the building into 'public' and 'work' zones. The general public are denied entry into the 'work' zone. Thus there is no access to the dispensary or areas used for storage other than for practice personnel. Medicines kept in the consulting rooms to which the public have access should be kept to a minimum, should not be drugs of abuse and should be kept in cupboards or drawers, not readily accessible to the client.

Well designed fixtures and fittings in areas where medicines are stored are necessary for efficient stock control and to reduce the possibility of-

a) breakage from over stocked shelves
b) accidents while stocking badly positioned shelves
c) contamination from unclean work surfaces

A dispensary should be fitted with a generous area of work bench which can be easily cleaned. Laminate is an ideal material for this purpose. Products in constant use should be readily accessible. Shelves should be sufficiently narrow to allow only one row of containers so that each preparation is visible. Sliding glass doors provide protection against accidental breakage and dust.

It is convenient to store medicines in the dispensary in logical groups such as antidiarrhoeals, anti inflammatories, antibiotics etc. It may be considered helpful to display tablets in the dispensary in uniform containers labelled with the name and strength of the drug, its unit retail price and number or colour coding to denote position on the shelf. Products such as injectables and ointments may also be colour coded and be labelled with a unit retail price.

Stable kick-stools should be provided. Products in larger containers should be stocked near to ground level. Injury may be incurred by personnel attempting to reach containers on shelves above head height.

Floors should be impervious, easy to clean and non slip. Terrazzo tiles and sheet vinyl are the materials most commonly used.

Security of the building
Sites for possible unlawful entry should be reduced to a minimum. No unnecessary windows should be constructed at the rear of new buildings; roof lights are more secure. Vulnerable windows may be fitted with toughened or wired glass or be protected with metal guards. Window frames should be strong and efficient to which locks may be fitted. Doors, particularly at the rear of the buildings, should be robust and have strong fittings and burglar alarms installed.

Night staff should ensure all door and windows are securely locked.

Fire precautions
Due to the highly flammable nature of some products (as well as reagents and other materials) it is advisable to have the premises inspected by a fire prevention officer from the local fire service. Advice will be given on the provision of fire extinguishers, fire doors and fire escapes. It is extremely important that smoking is prohibited in all areas where animal medicines are stored or used.

Storage conditions and temperatures
The heating, lighting and ventilation must be sufficient to provide a suitable storage temperature and humidity. Protection from the effects of sunlight and atmospheric moisture must be provided.

In purpose-built premises consideration should be given to incorporating at the outset an air-conditioning system set to run at a maximum of approximately 18°C.

Adequate refrigeration space must be provided. A large refrigerator may be necessary in the store room for bulk storage, with a smaller model in the dispensary or the consulting room for products in frequent use.

A refrigerator must run at 2°C to 8°C and should be fitted with some means for the regular daily monitoring and recording of temperatures, such as a maximum/minimum thermometer and a dedicated log book.

Regular (annual) recalibration or replacement of the maximum/minimum thermometer is essential as is the routine service and calibration (at least annually) of the refrigerator itself.

Since the completion of the product licence review of pharmaceutical products and with the ongoing licence review of biologicals, product labels now clearly state the licensed storage conditions and temperatures.

Broadly speaking vaccines and other biologicals are required to be stored between +2°C and +8°C.

Pharmaceuticals now specify the precise temperature limits, for example: 'Store up to 25°C. 'Do not freeze' is now commonly found on product labels.

However, it is important that product labels are reviewed periodically by a designated person within the practice and that the labels of all new product are carefully scrutinised.

Ventilation
Certain volatile agents such as ether and cyclopropane present a fire and explosion risk whilst agents such as halothane and organophosphates may be injurious to health. Wherever volatile compounds or aerosols are stored or used involving possible contamination of the atmosphere it is recommended that an adequate ventilation system is provided. Any ventilation system fitted should be capable of effecting a minimum of 10 air changes per hour.

Clean and Tidy
It is important for efficiency and maintenance of quality, safety and efficacy to ensure the dispensary and store rooms are kept clean and tidy.

MANAGEMENT
It is advisable for each practice to designate a veterinary surgeon to have overall responsibility for carrying out practice policy on storage, stock control, dispensing and safety.

Safety Policy
Under the Health and Safety at Work, etc Act 1974, all employers (of more than four employees) are obliged to provide their staff with a written statement of safety policy (see Chapter 3). The Act gives no guidance on what the policy should specify, except that the employer's general policy concerning health and safety at work of his employees should be given, together with arrangements made for carrying out that policy (eg the appointment of safety officers). The policy and any revision made to it must be brought to the attention of all employees. Such a policy could include information under the following headings where animal medicines are handled at work.

a. Dispensing or supply of animal medicines
b. Labelling of animal medicines
c. Prohibition of smoking (fire risk and transfer of drugs to the mouth by cigarettes etc)
d. Prohibition of eating, drinking and storage of human food in areas where medicinal products are stored or supplied
e. Hygiene
f. Handling of bulky or heavy packages
g. Emergency procedures to be adopted in the case of accident (this applies particularly to 'Immobilon'). The telephone numbers of doctors, hospitals, fire services and poison centres can be listed.

Standard Operating Procedures (SOP's)
Apart from the safety policy, practices should develop a manual of SOP's covering key activities and elements of the premises, facilities, equipment

and motor car. All employees should acknowledge receipt of their copy of the SOP's relevant to their function. The SOP's should be tested occasionally and reviewed periodically and employees advised of any changes.

Training
Staff training and re-training is important at all levels within the practice. A training policy should be prepared and a record kept of all training undertaken. Training for all employees working in the pharmacy and dispensary is essential and is now available through vocational organisations leading to formal qualifications, as well as from in-house personnel.

Stock control
In order to ensure efficiency, profitability, to reduce accidents and avoid abuse it is imperative that a practice adopts a good stock control system. An inventory should be drawn up of all the medicines in stock. Those that are of no further use because the expiry date has passed, or the product is no longer used by the practice, or containers are not identifiable, should be disposed of safely. A regular critical review should be made of all products used by the practice with special reference to controlled drugs.

Unless a product has an undoubted place in the practice no further order should be placed. In a similar way a critical appraisal should be made before any new product is stocked. A simple stock taking and re-ordering system should be adopted. Advice on available systems will normally be given by the wholesalers supplying the practice. A good system will minimize problems caused by overstocking, understocking or pilfering. To avoid the purchase of unnecessary products, or of duplication, it is advisable that all orders are checked by the designated senior member of staff.

All deliveries should be checked against delivery notes as soon as possible after arrival. A record of all deliveries should be kept, discrepancies noted and a system of correction implemented. Invoices should be checked by the designated member of staff.

Stock Returns
Manufacturers' and wholesalers' premises are strictly regulated by the Medicines Control Agency. However, once products have left these premises formal control of quality is lost. Therefore, over-ordering by a practice should be avoided and delivery discrepancies rapidly identified. Although immediate (same day or next day) return may be acceptable it is unreasonable to expect to be able to return in-date product which has been in the practice for some time in conditions outside the control of the supplier. This would generally be an unacceptable scenario to a practice which subsequently took delivery of that product.

Controlled Drugs

Under the Misuse of Drugs Act 1971 various dangerous drugs such as etorphine (Immobilon), morphine and cocaine are subject to particularly strict control. Such products present an attractive target not only to addicts but to professional criminals aware of large profits to be made from illicit drug sales. Advice should be obtained from the local Crime Prevention Officer on the suitability of premises, receptacles etc. for controlled drugs. It is important to note that

a. Schedule 2 controlled drugs must be kept in a locked receptacle which can only be opened by the veterinary surgeon or by a person authorised by him to do so. This is best implemented by having no more than one key to the receptacle per veterinary surgeon. The keys should be kept on the person.

b. A register must be kept of all Schedule 2 controlled drugs obtained, supplied or administered. Entries should be made within 24 hours of receipt or supply. A description of the requirements relating to the register has previously been described.

c. A locked car is not considered a locked receptacle within the meaning of the Misuse of Drugs (Safe Custody) Regulations.

d. Only the minimum quantity of controlled drugs should be stored

e. If etorphine (Immobilon) is to be stocked, then each practice must produce a clear statement for all personnel on the safest method of use of this highly toxic agent. The antidote (Narcan) and instructions for use in emergencies, must be carried with each container of 'Immobilon'.

Dispensing and supply

Veterinary surgeons are permitted to sell or supply POM, P and PML products only for animals under their care. GSL products may be supplied to anyone. Veterinary surgeons wishing to sell or supply PML products for animals not under their care must register as merchants. They must operate as a separate business and from premises separated from the veterinary practice. The special requirements for merchants are described in Chapter 1.

To avoid accidents from careless use, all medicines must be dispensed in suitable containers and must be clearly labelled (see Chapter 7).

Veterinary practices should have a clearly defined policy on the supply of medicines. Apart from GSL products, medicines should never be dispensed automatically or on demand. Preparations which may be dispensed by lay staff and those only to be dispensed by a veterinary surgeon must each be identified and no client should be supplied with a repeat prescription without the authority of a veterinary surgeon.

The principles governing which licensed drug may be used or dispensed for a particular species or purpose are defined in the so-called 'cascade' (see Chapter 7).

A record should be kept of all drugs that are dispensed.

Transportation (also see Chapter 6)
The motor car is a constant show-piece of the veterinary surgeon and the practice.

Care should be taken that medicines carried in veterinary surgeons' vehicles are kept at the conditions recommended by the manufacturers, particularly those relating to maximum and minimum temperature.

The car should be organised in a fixed way. Cross contamination must be prevented so drugs, instruments, equipment, empties, etc must be kept separate, with boots and disinfectant in a boot box and gowns in a special container.

Make a list of the drugs which are routinely necessary and stick to it and then only in small quantities!

All medicines should be well packed to avoid breakage.

Security should be given a high priority. A locked car is NOT considered to be a locked receptacle within the meaning of the Misuse of Drugs (Safe Custody) Regulations.

A drug inventory should be maintained for each practice vehicle and expiry dates noted.

A record should be kept of drug usage and hand-out of drugs.

More than one vial of an identical product should not be in use at the same time.

Write on each vial the date of first broaching. If the date of first use is in doubt, then discard.

In-car temperature control systems are now available for sensitive drugs and vaccines.

Set fixed times/dates for cleaning and reorganisation of the car boot area.

Summary
The manufacturer has obtained the licence (marketing authorisation) specifying the quality, safety and efficacy of a product. The label specifies the licensed storage conditions including temperature, humidity and light necessary to maintain licensed quality up to the stated expiry date. The data sheet specifies other conditions such as: reconstitution requirements for vaccines, duration of use of part-used vials, whether products may be mixed for use etc, as well as route, dose and contra-indications. Compromising any of these conditions is likely to compromise the licensed quality, safety and efficacy of a product.

Chapter 6

Transport of Animal Medicines

Roger R Cook & Stephen Dawson

For the majority of persons involved in transporting licensed animal medicines, the product is in clean, sealed packs and so the concern is with the potential hazard which might result from an "incident" such as breakage during loading or unloading, or a road accident.

Much of the action necessitated by transport regulations will be the responsibility of the product manufacturer, who has to ensure that the packaging of a product complies with the regulations. Nevertheless they are summarised below to provide background and assist understanding.

For those in the supply chain "downstream" from the manufacturer the key areas are:
- to understand the meaning of the various warning diamonds on transport packs, and to be aware of the action necessary in the event of an incident involving each class of hazard.
- to ensure that drivers of vehicles have the necessary information to respond to incidents involving the products they are carrying at any time
- where activity involves the opening of combination packs to create mixed consignments, to ensure that the assembled consignment is suitably packaged to protect against any transport incident.

If in doubt, the user should ask the supplier whether the product is dangerous for carriage. If a pack is bought as supplied by the manufacturer, then the labelling should make this clear. However, the manufacturer may not label the inner packs, so it is important to check that these are also safe for independent transport.

(Eventually advice on meeting these responsibilities should become available from specially designated "Dangerous Goods Advisors".)

There is a variety of legislation relating to the transport of chemicals and other goods, but from the point of view of the user of animal medicines, the major regulations are the CDG(CPL) regulations. (Other regulations deal with transport in tankers, of explosives etc.)

CDG(CPL) Transport Regulations
The Carriage of Dangerous Goods by Road and Rail (Classification, Packaging and Labelling) Regulations 1994 (S.I. 1994/669) came into force on 1 April 1994. These replace previous legislation[1] and implement part of EC Directive 94/55/EC (sometimes known as the ADR (Agreement concerning the international carriage of Dangerous goods by Road) Framework Directive), bringing legislation into line with the UN Recommendations on the Transport of Dangerous Goods. They also extend legislation to rail transport (previously covered by British Rail's conditions of acceptance). These Regulations are concerned with the transport of dangerous goods, and are aimed at ensuring the health and safety of those involved with, or liable to be affected by, their transport.

One significant change is that medicines are no longer exempted, since government felt that the Medicines Act and related legislation was directed towards safe use of goods, and that considerations are different when transportation is involved. Another important difference is that the cut-off for toxicity is higher for transport than for use, because the transport regulations are not concerned with long term low level exposure. In transport, the potential immediate hazard of a particular substance is the prime consideration, and so information on, for example, its flammability or toxicity, must be available in a form which is readily understood by those involved in transport or responding to a transport incident.

If the Regulations apply, then the product must be in "type approved" packaging, and the label must show the appropriate transport hazard diamond(s) and UN number. However, it is likely that many veterinary medicines will not be caught by the Regulations, either because of their low intrinsic hazard or the small pack size.

Pack type
Having decided that the product is "dangerous", the next step is to consider the pack itself. The product is allocated to one of the following Packing Groups, where the size is the receptacle in contact with the dangerous good, e.g. if it is a bubble pack, the individual bubble is considered.

I. so dangerous that there is no minimum size, e.g. cytotoxins, anaesthetics
II. size not exceeding 500g for solids, 100ml for liquids
III. size not exceeding 3kg for solids, 5kg for liquids

Aerosols are classed by volume of carrier/propellant plus product.

The pack must be of an approved type, with the testing looking at durability and general safety and suitability for transport.

There is a wide variety of type-approved packaging available. All goods imported or exported already require it, as do products moved by sea (Northern Ireland, Isle of Wight, etc) so in many cases no change to previous procedures is needed.

Limited Quantities

In determining whether a product pack is hazardous, both the product itself and the size of the pack must be considered. Products classified as dangerous for transport and in pack sizes smaller than those in the Limited Quantity provisions (Schedule 3 of the Regulations) need not be packaged and labelled according to the Regulations. For example, a corrosive solid in Packing Group II may be transported in packs up to 2kg without restriction under the Regulations. Products in bubble packs will not be deemed hazardous, since the individual bubble is considered as the pack size.

If the gross mass of the package does not exceed 30kg, UN type-approval is not required provided that the individual pack capacity does not exceed the limit set down in Schedule 3. The packaging must merely be "of good quality, fit for the purpose". A simple designation is required on the pack, together with the UN number.

Transitional Arrangements

By anticipating the parts of the ADR Framework Directive concerning the classification, packaging and labelling of dangerous goods, the UK government was able to take advantage of a concession in the Directive whereby changes would not be required to domestic requirements which were already totally aligned with the worldwide UN Recommendations for the Carriage of Dangerous Goods. This was felt to be particularly important since the UK regulations were much closer to the UN Recommendations than the ADR. Since the UN Recommendations are not quite so restrictive and prescriptive as ADR's requirements, and in some cases less so than previous British legislation, costs to industry may be reduced.

The Regulations provide transitional arrangements to try to meet some of industry's concerns:

- Goods packed and labelled according to the previous arrangements (even if the previous arrangements did not impose any particular requirements) prior to 1 July 1995 may be shipped to their final destination until 31 December 1998.

- Packaging purchased before 1 July 1995 may be used, providing that the manufacturing date is clearly stated on the pack. These packs must reach their final destination by 1 January 1999. (The requirement that the packaging should be less than five years old at final delivery has been removed by the HSE certificate of exemption (No. 6 of 1995), with the exception of plastic drums and jerrycans.)

Combination Packs

A combination pack consists of an outer transport carton which contains a number of smaller packs. Problems arise when these combination packs are split. For example, a vet might split a pack to put individual bottles in his car for his rounds, or a farmer could transport bottles to the farm. This could be an offence, since even though the combination pack complies with the new Regulations, the individual inner pack may not. In practice, though, small size and low hazard mean that many inner packs do not require type-approved packaging.

In the past, the inner packs had difficulties passing the stacking test. An improved UK interpretation of the UN recommendations means that bottles no longer need to be stackable, but merely to support load. This may increase the number of inners which are type-approved, and so can be moved on their own.

The Health and Safety Executive have issued an exemption certificate (No. 3 of 1995) to allow the use and purchase until 31 December 1995 of combination packs with non-approved inner packs for Packing Groups II and III up to a maximum inner pack size of 5 litres. This will be reviewed at the end of the year. HSE have said that it might be extended if there is evidence that efforts have been made to seek alternative UN type approved packaging but that more time is needed. It is unlikely that this exemption will last indefinitely since the UN Regulations define the maximum as 1 litre.

At the time of writing (October 1995), HSE has said that after representations from manufacturers, it is extremely likely that this will be extended for another six months.

From the point of view of the user, a problem this generates is that the current exemption limits use to six months. Therefore inners from combination packs which are currently exempted may not be transported individually after 31 December 1995. HSE recognises this problem and has promised to address it in the proposed extension to the exemption certificate.

Mixed Dangerous Goods in Limited Quantities
HSE has issued an indefinite certificate of exemption (No. 4 of 1995), reducing the labelling requirements for single packages containing mixed dangerous goods in limited quantities (i.e. those laid down by Schedule 3). This would apply, for example, to a container with several different bottles. The certificate permits simplified labelling, allowed internationally, by either

- following the International Maritime Dangerous Goods (IMDG) Code system for the labelling of limited quantities of mixed goods, or
- marking the packages with the United Nations number(s) (preceded by the letters UN) of the products contained within a package.

The Future

Dangerous Goods Advisers
The EC has issued a draft directive, expected to become law within the next twelve months, proposing that by 1 January 2000, undertakings whose activities include the transport of dangerous goods appoint one or more safety advisers on the transport of dangerous goods, responsible for helping to safeguard against the risks inherent in those activities with regard to public safety, property and the environment.

This safety adviser will have to hold a vocational training certificate, valid for the modes of transport involved (as is already the case for transportation by sea or air). Anything classed as dangerous under the CDG(CPL) Regulations is likely to be affected, and there is currently no minimum size of "undertaking" which is required to comply. However it seems probable that the adviser can be an external consultant rather than a company employee.

Further changes
Additional changes are on the way. It is planned to release a consultative document on regulations to implement the rest of the ADR Directive on 30 November 1995. It is the current intention to harmonise ADR and the UN Recommendations, but it is possible that in the future the EC could decide to end the concession allowing the retention of domestic arrangements which meet the UN Recommendations.

Notes
[1] The CDG (CPL) regulations replace the road carriage provisions in the Chemicals (Hazard Information and Packaging) Regulations 1993 (CHIP).

Chapter 7

Dispensing, Labelling and Manufacturers' Instructions

P D Simm revised by Dr Michael H Jepson

Introduction
The number and complexity of animal medicines which are available to the veterinary surgeon, farmer, horse and pet owners have steadily increased, and it is important that all medicinal products are dispensed, labelled and used correctly.

The requirements for dispensing and labelling animal medicines are defined in detail in various Orders and Statutory Instruments (SIs) made under the Medicines Act 1968, and these apply not only to manufacturers but in part to all those concerned in the distribution of medicinal products.

The veterinarian, pharmacist, animal health distributor, and feed compounder should not only comply with the regulations but should also take responsibility for generating an awareness on the part of the end user as to the manner in which animal medicines should be stored, handled and administered. Any unused medication must be disposed of safely and legally.

The following sections must only be regarded as a summary of the more important aspects. A comprehensive review of dispensing and labelling requirements can be made by reference to the various orders, some of which are listed at the end of this chapter, or by reference to the Law Department of the Royal Pharmaceutical Society of Great Britain or to the Veterinary Medicines Directorate.

Dispensing
'Dispensed' animal medicines are those supplied by a veterinary surgeon or in accordance with a prescription given by him. The term also applies to certain medicinal products that are exempt from licensing requirements under the Medicines Act 1968, when prepared or supplied from a registered pharmacy at the request of the purchaser.

It should be noted that although a pharmacist, on request, may use his own judgement as to the treatment required (from the range of products that are not restricted to prescription) this only applies where the treatment is for human use. A pharmacist is not allowed to make a diagnosis of animal's condition; counter-prescribing for an animal patient is not permissible under the Veterinary Surgeons Act 1966. When a medicine is requested for treatment based on the diagnosis of the purchaser, eg, a request for a treatment for fluke or scour, a pharmacist may at his discretion prescribe or supply any licensed product with that indication for use, that is not restricted to supply on prescription (see Chapter 1).

Relatively few animal medicines today are prepared in veterinary practice or in pharmacies, the majority of dispensed medicines are manufactured on a large scale by the pharmaceutical industry as proprietary or generic products.

The key to good dispensing practice is the correct and safe interpretation of the wishes of the prescriber. Where a proprietary product is prescribed the product should be supplied in its original pack with an appropriate dispensing label (see later) attached, so as not to obscure any important printed information on the manufacturers' label or pack. Package inserts or leaflets must not be removed.

New Administration Regulations introduced on 31 December 1994, implement the European Community Directive 90/676 and replace the 1983 Regulations (SI 1994 No. 2987 Medicines (Restriction of Veterinary Medicinal Products) Regulations 1994). The Regulations establish in law the 'cascade' and control the prescription by veterinarians of veterinary medicinal products of all legal categories for animals under their care, whether food-producing or companion animals.

When no authorised veterinary medicinal product exists for a condition in a particular species, and in order to avoid causing unacceptable suffering, veterinary surgeons exercising their clinical judgement may prescribe for one or a small number of animals under their care in accordance with the following sequence:

(i)   a veterinary medicine authorised for use in another species, or for a different use in the same species ('off-label use');
(ii) a medicine authorised in the UK for human use;
(iii) a medicine to be made up at the time on a one-off basis by a veterinary surgeon or a properly authorised person.
(for further information see AMELIA 8, as mentioned in 'further information' section of this chapter, also Chapter 12).

Consideration must be given to repack the preparation (unless this is not possible, eg, a sterile product) in a suitable container labelled according to the directions given in the prescription.

Animal medicines may be dispensed from bulk supplies by a veterinary surgeon or practitioner, and by a pharmacist. Animal health distributors may not break bulk (see Chapter 1).

Containers
Preparations dispensed from bulk packs should be supplied in suitable containers. Tablets and capsules should be placed in airtight containers made of light resistant glass, metal (aluminimum) or rigid plastic. Liquid preparations for oral administration should be dispensed in amber glass, or suitable rigid plastic bottles. Semi-solid preparations should be packed in ointment jars.

Liquid animal medicines for external use containing one or more of the substances listed in the schedule to SI 1978 No. 40 must be placed in a fluted bottle (vertically ribbed so as to be discernible by touch)[2].

This requirement does not apply to containers of a capacity greater than 1.14 litres or to eye or ear-drops supplied in plastic containers. 'External use' in relation to animal medicines means application to the skin, hair, fur, feathers, scales, hoof, horn, ear, eye, mouth or mucosa of the throat or prepuce.

(Veterinarians and pharmacists should dispense medicines in child resistant containers unless they are supplied in foil or strip packaging.)

Cardboard boxes can be used as secondary packaging for tablets or capsules contained in foil or strip packaging. Envelopes are not good practice and should not be used.

Records
There is no legal necessity for a veterinarian to keep a record of the medicinal products he supplies or dispenses, except in the case of a Schedule 2 controlled drug register (see Chapter 2). However it is recommended that a record should be kept in the practice of drugs allowed to be supplied to particular farms.

The record should be signed by the veterinarian who has the animals under his or her care. Each POM order dispensed should be signed by the veterinarian or member of the lay staff, acting under the supervision of the veterinarian who dispenses the product. Under no circumstances should prescriptions or POMs supplied by a pharmacist be changed without the permission of the responsible veterinarian.

Pharmacists must retain prescriptions for prescription only medicines for two years from the date of supply and enter the particulars in a Prescription Only Register[4].

Animal health distributors are required to keep records of sales of Merchants' List (PML) products for two years from the date of supply. The date of sale, the name, quantity, form and strength of the preparation supplied, and the name and address of the purchaser must be recorded.

It is good practice to record the batch numbers of drugs supplied to assist in cases of re-call or complaint.

Labelling

The labelling requirements for medicinal products are given in regulations made under the Medicines Act 1968[1,5]. The only regulations that are described here apply to dispensed medicinal products.

'Dispensed medicinal products' are defined for the purposes of the labelling regulations as medicines which are either:

(i) prepared or dispensed in accordance with a prescription given by a doctor, dentist or veterinary surgeon or practitioner (or prepared or dispensed by the practitioner), or

(ii) sold or supplied by a doctor or dentist for administration to a particular patient of his (or in the case of veterinary medicines sold or supplied by a veterinary surgeon or practitioner for administration to a particular animal or herd which is under his care), or

(iii) prepared or dispensed in registered pharmacy by or under the supervision of a pharmacist in the circumstances set out in Section 10(3) (specification furnished by the purchaser) or Section 10(4) (a) (pharmacist's own judgement) of the Medicines Act 1968, or

(iv) sold or supplied to a particular person who has specifically requested the person selling or supplying the product to use his own judgement as to the treatment required. (NB: this does not apply in the case of animal medicines for the reasons given earlier in the chapter under 'Dispensing').

Labelling of dispensed animal medicines

In preference the container of the dispensed animal medicines, or failing that the outer package, must be labelled in an indelible manner, with the following particulars: (NB: if the product contains hexachlorophane BOTH the container and the package must be labelled with warnings as under 7).

1. The name of the person who has possession or control of the animal or herd, and the address of the premises where the animal or herd is kept, or the address of one such premises.
2. The name and address of the veterinarian.
3. The date of dispensing.

4. The words 'for animal treatment only' - unless the container or package is too small for it to be reasonably practicable to do so.
5. The words 'keep out of the reach of children' or words with a similar meaning.
6. The words 'for external use only' for medicines that are only for topical use, such as if the product is an embrocation, liniment, lotion, liquid antiseptic or other liquid preparation or gel.
7. If the product contains hexachlorophane and is for oral administration for the prevention or treatment of fluke disease in sheep and cattle; a warning that protective clothing must be worn by the operator when the product is being administered. If such a product is for cattle: an additional warning that the product is not for use in lactating cows. Both container and outer packaging should be labelled.
8. The relevant withdrawal period should always be stated on medicinal products for food-producing animals, even if nil.

Where appropriate, precautions relating to the use of the product to ensure operator safety.

Two practical examples are shown in Figure 1.

Figure 1

Example 1 Dispensing 20 x 10mg Ace promazine tablets for a dog.

Legally required	For Animal Treatment Only For Mrs Smith's dog (name) 8 Long Lane, Coxton, Surrey 28/7/95
Recommended	20 Ace promazine tables 10mg Two* 0.25-3 mg/kg tablets to be given by mouth before food for preventing travel sickness
Legally required	Keep all medicines out of reach of children J G BLOGGS, MRCVS Veterinary Surgeon 2 High Street, Coxton, Surrey

Example 2 Dispensing Framycetin Injection 15% for a cow.

Legally required	For Animal Treatment Only For F Giles Cow, No. 343 Ash Farm, Coxton, Surrey 28/7/95
Recommended	100ml Framycetin Injection 15% w/v Framycetin sulphate 150mg in 1ml 1ml per 30kg bodyweight* by intramuscular injection twice daily for not more than 3 days FOR INTRAMUSCULAR USE ONLY Milk must not be used for human consumption during treatment Once broached use within 3 weeks Withdrawal periods: cattle: slaughter 49 days, milk 72 hours (3 days)(7 milkings) Store below 15°C (do not freeze). Expiry date........
Legally required	Keep all medicines out of reach of children. J G BLOGGS, MRCVS Veterinary Surgeon 2 High Street, Coxton, Surrey

*May be more appropriate to give actual dose for individual animal

NOTE: The information shown as 'recommended', is not strictly legally required, but its omission could be considered professionally irresponsible and negligent especially in the event of unsafe use.

For medicinal products, such as the injection illustrated in Example 2, it is important to avoid any obscuring of the manufacturer's label. The information will include the marketing authorisation (product licence) and batch numbers, expiry date and any special storage requirements, any special warnings and legal classification.

The manufacturer's information will also include the species of animal for which the product is intended and licensed, as well as the withdrawal periods required where products are intended for administration to food-producing animals.

If a veterinarian prescribes a medicine, he may request that it be labelled with any of the following particulars (which he would, if he were dispensing direct to the client himself, draw specifically to the client's attention):

(a) the name of the product
(b) directions for use
(c) precautions relating to the use of the product

If a pharmacist dispensing such a prescription considers that any of the requested particulars a, b or c are inappropriate and is unable to contact the veterinarian, he has the professional discretion to substitute other particulars of the same kind to ensure the safety of the patient and administrator. Additional information can also be given.

The labelling requirements apply whether the medicines are dispensed in the manufacturer's original container or dispensed from bulk into smaller packs.

Although appropriate labels can be ordered from any printer, there are firms specialising in their production who advertise in the professional journals (eg The Veterinary Record).

'For animal treatment only' must be included on the label of every veterinary drug and every leaflet supplied with a veterinary drug. The only exemption is if the container or package to be labelled is so small that it is not reasonably practicable to show such words.

Medicinal products and medicated feedingstuffs

The container and package of a dispensed medicinal product for incorporation in animal feeding stuffs, or which is a medicated animal feeding stuff in respect of which a product licence has been granted, must be labelled with the following particulars:

1. The particulars required for a dispensed medicinal product must be as described under 1-8 above AND
2. Additional information required under Section 14(3) of the regulations that are set out in Schedule 4 to the regulations; as amended.

NOTE: The additional information required in 2 above will appear on the manufacturer's label.

Where the licensed feed additive or medicated feed is supplied by the manufacturer in a container that is too small to accommodate all the information required of him this must be supplied in an accompanying leaflet. This is also applicable where the licensed product is not supplied in containers for bulk feed.

Product instructions
Product information is supplied by the marketing authorisation or product licence holder of an animal medicine or medicinal feed additive on the container and packs, package insert leaflets, and data sheets. To make appropriate and safe use of the product the directions given should be followed implicitly.

Label information
Marketing authorisation or product licence holders are required to ensure that animal medicines are labelled in accordance with the labelling regulations made under the Medicines Act 1968[5]. The regulations, as they apply to the manufacturer, are detailed and are not described here. Attention is drawn however, to the following information given on the labels and/or packs of animal medicines.

Directions for use: Directions for use and the purpose(s) for which the animal medicine is to be used will be given. (These may not be given if the product is only available on prescription or is not supplied by retail in the manufacturer's container.) It is important that these are followed. The species of animal for which the drug is intended. A veterinarian, for example, who does not follow a marketing authorisation holder's instructions or uses a product for a purpose other than that indicated by the marketing authorisation holder does so entirely at his own professional risk without recourse to the marketing authorisation holder (see earlier section on the 'cascade').

Dosage: The optimal effects of many medicines are achieved on a strict mg per kg bodyweight basis, yet weight is rarely measured prior to dosing. Under or over dosing is probably the rule rather than the exception. Particularly when changing brands, dosage must be redefined, as Brand A may contain twice the concentration of active ingredient of Brand B and therefore require a much lower dosage regime.

Route of administration: Particular care should be taken to observe the recommended route of dosing. Injectable products may be designed for specific routes only - eg intravenous, intramuscular, or subcutaneous.

Precautions in use/contra-indications: This area is one which is frequently abused and many users of animal medicines continue not to 'wear gloves during an application' or to 'wash hands after use', or to apply other specified protective measures despite clear instructions to do so (see Chapters 4 and 13).

Withdrawal Period: which is mandatory before a treated animal is slaughtered for the production of food and before products derived from a treated animal are used as food.

Withdrawal period statements: A withdrawl period for an animal medicine is fixed by the Licensing Authority based on safety considerations. It should not be assumed that adherence to the withholding time will automatically satisfy the requirements of third parties (eg the sensitive Milk Marque tests for antibiotic residues in milk; for horse products, Jockey Club rules).

Expiry date: Where an animal medicine is to be used within three years of manufacture, an expiry date will, by law, be given on the container and pack. In practice, the VMD expects all products to have an expiry date regardless of the three year period. Products should not be used after the expiry date given.

Batch reference: A batch reference will be given on the container and package of the product. The letters 'BN' or 'LOT' will often precede the batch number. These letters will be omitted on small containers and certain collapsible tubes. The batch reference must be quoted in connection with any complaint concerning the quality of a product and should be recorded in any relevant records (see Chapter 13).

Additional note on Withdrawal Periods. When prescribing a veterinary product for a food-producing animal without the recommendations specified on the data sheet (that is, different dosage or for non-target species) or if the data sheet does not specify a withdrawal period the following minimum standard withdrawal periods should be observed:

Eggs	7 days
Milk	7 days
Meat[a] from poultry and mammals	28 days
Meat from fish	500 degree days[b]

[a] includes muscle, fat, liver, etc
[b] cumulative sum of mean daily water temperatures in degrees Celsius following the last treatment.

Package insert leaflets

Package insert leaflets are often supplied by the marketing authorisation holder to supplement the information given on the container and package of an animal medicine. These will often give similar information to that included on the Data Sheet (see below) which will be of use to the prescriber, distributor and the end user. As already mentioned, it is important that these leaflets do not become separated from the primary container, when the outer packs are split and supplied or dispensed by veterinarians or pharmacists.

Data sheets

The Medicines Act 1968 requires that, before sending or delivering an advertisement for an animal medicine to a veterinary surgeon or practitioner, or making an oral representation to him concerning the product, a Data Sheet must be sent or delivered to him describing and giving the essential particulars of the product, within the previous 15 months[6].

The contents of a Data Sheet are controlled by regulations made under the Medicines Act 1968[7]. Many pharmaceutical companies produce their own compendia or contribute to 'joint' Data Sheet compendia that are sent to practising veterinary surgeons and practitioners. An example of a 'joint' compendium is the NOAH Compendium of Data Sheets for Veterinary Products which is updated every fifteen months.

The Data Sheets for an animal medicine should be regarded as the standard reference for the product concerned. Additional information may be available on request from the marketing authorisation (product licence) holder.

Due Diligence

It is a defence under the Regulations for a person to prove that he or she took all reasonable precautions and exercised all due diligence to avoid the commission of an offence by him or herself or by someone acting under his or her direction. What precautions are reasonable would depend on the circumstances. For veterinarians the standard for due diligence would be that expected of a person of his or her professional standing.

Notes

1. VMD Guidance Note: AMELIA 4 (January 1995) Marketing Authorisations for Veterinary Medicinal Products: Requirements for Labels and Package Inserts.
2. Medicines (Fluted bottle) Regulations 1978, SI 1978 No. 40.
3. Medicines (Pharmacy and General Sale - Exemption) Order 1980, SI No. 1924
4. The Medicines (Sale or Supply)(Miscellaneous Provisions)Regulations1980, SI 1980 No. 1923.
5. The Medicines (Labelling) Regulations 1976 - SI 1976 No. 1726 as amended by: The Medicines (Labelling) Amendment Regulations to date.

For an interpretation of the principal labelling regulations as amended, see reference 1.
6. Section 96 of the Medicines Act 1968.
7. The Medicines (Data Sheet) Regulations 1972 - SI 1972 No. 2076. As amended by The Medicines (Data Sheet) Amendment Regulations 1981 - SI 1981 No. 1633; SI 1989 No. 1183.

Chapter 8

Sterility and Sterile Products

J E Brown revised by Dr John Dowrick

A sterile product is one in which all viable micro-organisms have been eliminated or excluded during manufacture.

Pharmaceutical products intended for injection, instillation into the eye or infusion into the teat canal must be sterile to stop the introduction of pathogenic organisms into body tissues. The following products are commonly used in veterinary medicine.

Eye drops
Eye drops are sterile solutions or suspensions of one or more drugs for instillation into the conjunctival sac.

Eye drops can contain drugs with antibacterial, anaesthetic, anti-inflammatory, miotic or mydriatic properties. The vehicle may be either aqueous or oily. Eye drops are supplied in multidose containers or in single dose packs. Multidose preparations contain, if necessary, preservative to ensure the product is protected from microbial contamination once the pack is opened. Products intended for single application do not contain a preservative. Eye drugs are manufactured and filled aseptically and are available in plastic containers fitted with a nozzle and screw cap.

Eye ointments
Eye ointments are sterile semi-solid preparations containing drug substances similar to eye drops. They are for application to the conjunctival sac. Suitable bases for eye ointments are paraffins which are heated to sterilise and solidify on cooling. The drug substance is aseptically suspended in the cooled base or dissolved in the molten paraffin before cooling.

Eye ointments are normally dispensed in sterile collapsible aluminium or plastic laminate tubes with screw caps.

Implants
Implants are sterile discs or cylinders containing drug substances. They are implanted in the body tissues either during minor surgery or by the use of an applicator. The drug substance is released at a controlled rate over a period of time. Implants are usually packed singly in sealed sterile tubes.

Injections

Injections are sterile solutions, suspensions or emulsions containing one or more drug substances in an aqueous or non-aqueous vehicle. They are used to administer drugs into the body tissues in cases where they are either therapeutically inactive or not tolerated when given orally. They are also used to administer drugs required to product a rapid, localised, or prolonged therapeutic effect, or immunological response, and additionally for many species are easier to administer.

Preparations intended for parenteral administration are manufactured using aseptic techniques thus eliminating the risk of introducing microbial contamination. Wherever possible injections are terminally sterilised in the final sealed container.

Injections are available in single dose and multidose containers - single dose preparations must be discarded after the one use. Multidose preparations normally contain an antimicrobial preservative which will ensure the sterility of the preparation for more than one use.

Single dose preparations are supplied in hermetically sealed ampoules. Multidose preparations are generally supplied in glass vials sealed with a rubber plug to allow easy withdrawal of doses.

Drug substances which are unstable in liquid form for any length of time are supplied as dry powders for constitution with a suitable diluent immediately prior to use. Such preparations are more widely used in human medicine than in veterinary practice. Infusion fluids are apyrogenic, sterile aqueous solutions or emulsions which have been rendered isotonic with blood. Infusion fluids do not contain preservatives.

Sterile dusting powders

Sterile dusting powders are generally applied to small wounds. They may contain fly repellents, antibacterial, antibiotic or haemostatic drug substances. Dusting powders are appropriately sterilised and are packed in multidose plastic puffer bottles.

Intramammary Infusions

Intramammary infusions are sterile suspensions of one or more drug substances, normally antibiotic, usually contained in an oily vehicle. They are intended for infusion into the teat canal.

There are two types of intramammary infusion available.
1. for lactating cows and
2. for dry cows

The product intended for the therapeutic treatment of mastitis in the lactating cow is formulated to provide effective antibiotic levels in the udder and a rapid 'milk out' time thus minimising the milk withholding time necessary to prevent residues in milk.

The dry cow product is formulated as a long acting preparation thus providing a persistent effective concentration of antibiotic in the udder for eliminating existing infections and preventing new infections during the dry period.

Intramammary infusions are supplied in single dose containers, normally a plastic syringe and nozzle fitted with a plastic cap. The smooth round nozzle facilitates insertion into the teat canal.

Avoidance of contamination
Great care has been taken to exclude micro-organisms from the product during manufacture.

For this reason it is critical that due care is taken to ensure there is little or no risk of accidentally contaminating a sterile product.

This is occasionally a problem in animal treatment as the farm environment may not be conducive to the maintenance of sterility.

Injectable products contained in multidose vials are sealed with a rubber plug seal to enable easy withdrawal of doses. Each time a dose is withdrawn the product is potentially at risk from the introduction of micro organisms. For this reason a sterile needle and syringe should be used for each withdrawal. The period of time between withdrawal of the first and last dose, which should be in accordance with the label instructions.

Eye drops and eye ointments supplied in multidose packs may potentially be at risk from the introduction of micro-organisms. Care must be exercised when administering the product to ensure the nozzle on the bottle or tube is not inadvertently touched by the operator and that infection is not passed from eye to eye or between animals.

It is important to observe the precautions recommended by the manufacturer when storing opened packs of products intended for multidose application. If in doubt any residue should be discarded. The effective cleaning of the teats and udder prior to the introduction of an intramammary infusion is critical in the avoidance of contamination and so enhances the success of treatment. Once the protective cap has been removed from the intramammary syringe, care must be taken to avoid accidentally contaminating the nozzle before insertion into the teat canal.

Further information on sterility and sterile products may be obtained from the British Pharmacopoeia. When using any animal medicine it is essential to follow the detailed instructions on the product label and on data sheets as well as these general guidelines.

Chapter 9

Antibiotics

A B Marshall revised by Dr Robin Bywater

An antibiotic is generally defined as a chemical substance provided wholly or partially by a micro organism (usually a fungus or bacterium) which has the capacity in dilute solution to inhibit the growth of, or to destroy bacteria and other micro organisms[1].

In this chapter, the term 'antibiotic' will include those chemical compounds (eg sulphonamides, nitrofurans, etc) which do not satisfy the above definition but nevertheless exhibit similar antimicrobial properties.

Storage

(a) **Temperature**

The majority of antibiotic preparations should be stored in a cool place (below 25°C), although some need to be refrigerated (2-8°C). High storage temperatures will accelerate chemical decomposition and shorten the shelf life of the product.

Very low temperatures should be avoided for similar reasons (eg ampicillin sodium in solution shows a greater loss of potency between -20°C and 0°C than if just refrigerated).

The particle size of suspensions may increase as a result of fluctuating storage temperatures, which can affect drug bio-availability due to a reduction in surface area of the suspended solid.

The boot of a car is a particularly unsuitable environment for the storage of animal medicines. In summer, temperatures can reach 40°C or more, falling to below zero in winter. Only such stock as will be used in the immediate future should be kept in the car.

Oily suspensions, including oral dosers, intramammary and intrauterine infusions, and some injectables may require warming to not more than room temperature before use simply because the cold suspension is too viscous to easily pass through a pump, cannula or needle.

(b) **Moisture**

Tablets, capsules and powders are often adversely affected by moisture, and should be kept in their original containers, the lid being properly replaced after use. Partly used sachets should be discarded since the protection provided by this form of packaging will have been destroyed on opening, and a rapid loss of antibiotic potency may ensue.

Desiccants, in small porous packs, are sometimes inserted amongst tablets and capsules to protect them from moisture. These should be retained wherever possible.

Certain antibiotics (eg Penicillin G) are unstable in water even for short periods of time, and are presented in dry powder form for reconstitution with water (sterile or otherwise, as directed), immediately before use.

Antibiotic sensitivity discs should be stored in a refrigerator but the container must be warmed to room temperature before opening, to avoid condensation on the internal walls of the vessel.

(c) **Light**
Antibiotic solutions (eg streptomycin, neomycin and the tetracyclines) can be affected by light. Some solutions may darken on exposure to light, although there may be little loss of potency.

In some cases, exposure to light causes decomposition as well as colour change. Solutions or suspensions showing marked discolouration should not be used as the potency of the preparation will be uncertain.

Antibiotic preparations are often stored under unsuitable conditions on the farm. For example: products stored on the window ledge in the milking parlour (often the only 'shelf' available) are exposed to direct sunlight, wide temperature variation, moisture, and to possible contamination with dung and dust. A simple cupboard, protected from extremes of temperature, and out of reach of children and animals, will satisfy the storage requirements for most products.

(d) **Vibration**
The physical stability of tablets, capsules, and suspensions can be adversely affected by mechanical vibration encountered in transit. Tablets may chip, fracture or powder. The headspace in bottles or containers is usually filled with a foam or cotton wool wad to protect the tablets or capsules during transport. Tablets or capsules that will be stored in the car should be prevented from rattling by the retention of the wadding.

(e) **Shelf Life**
Antibiotic preparations are often relatively unstable, and are given an expiry date after which they should be discarded. The shelf life is determined by the manufacturer storing the product at various temperatures and humidities, and is commonly the time taken for the potency of the preparation to fall to 90 per cent of the nominal potency.

The importance of an efficient stock control system cannot be over emphasised. Incoming stock must not be used until existing stocks have been exhausted.

Handling
Antibiotic compounds may occasionally bring about an allergic response caused by the routine handling of preparations containing these materials. Contact by the handler must be minimised and it is particularly advisable to wash hands after the use of an antibiotic product.

Where powders are handled, care should be taken to avoid the inhalation of dust from the product. A suitable form of dust mask should be worn especially where large quantities of powder are involved.

The aminoglycosides (eg streptomycin, neomycin, framycetin) may cause contact dermatitis in sensitised individuals. Sensitisation may be brought about just by handling the product.

Contact with penicillin or cephalosporins may also cause sensitisation. Veterinary surgeons, veterinary nurses, pharmacists and some farmers handle antibiotic preparations daily and over a period of many years. To suffer from an antibiotic allergy in such occupations is an inconvenience which can be avoided by minimising direct contact and by careful handling.

Dispensing and administration
Before the treatment of an animal patient with an antibiotic preparation the following points should be considered:-

Suspensions
The container must be shaken well to ensure an even dispersion. This does not just mean removing the caked material from the bottom of the bottle but means enough shaking to ensure that the sediment completely breaks up. A well formulated product should resuspend easily. If this is not done with multi-dose containers the patient may receive mainly vehicle and very little of the active constituent (eg with oral dosers and suspensions for injection) or vice-versa.

Dispensing
Whenever medicines are dispensed from a bulk supply for an individual animal a suitable new container must be used which MUST be labelled immediately in accordance with current Labelling Regulations (see Chapter 7). The suitability of a container will depend on the light and moisture stability of the product and the length of time before the final dose will be used. The headspace of vials and ampoules may have been filled with an inert gas to protect against oxidation. This protection is lost as soon as the first dose is removed.

Paper envelopes have been widely used for tablets and capsules in the past but these provide little physical or moisture protection and should not be used.

Sterility
Antibiotic preparations for other than oral or most topical use are manufactured under aseptic conditions. They must be used in a manner that ensures they remain free from contamination. It is recommended that intramammary tubes and syringes should only be inserted into the cow's teat after it has been thoroughly swabbed with surgical spirit or a similar agent. Sterile syringes and needles must be used with injectable products.

Multi-dose antibiotic injection vials pose a special problem since the rubber bung is breached as the first dose is removed. Even though the vial contains antibiotic, the contents can become contaminated with micro organisms that are unaffected by that compound. For this reason multi-dose formulations usually contain preservatives (eg benzalkonium chloride, chlorocresol), to ensure they are self sterilising. The aim must to be swab the cap prior to inserting the needle, to always use a sterile syringe and needle, and to finish such bottles within a reasonable time, in accordance with label instructions as to when to discard any remaining product.

Syringes
The choice of syringe type is important with some oily injections. Ethyl oleate is a common vehicle for oily formulations which may be incompatible with polystyrene syringes. Poly-propylene syringes should be used on these occasions. Oil based formulations often remove the silicone lubricant from the syringe barrel, and so increase resistance to plunger movement. This effect varies between different manufacturers' syringes.

Drug incompatabilities
If two or more products are mixed together prior to administration they may react with each other with detrimental results.

As a general rule, if two drugs are being injected at the same time, they should not be mixed together in the syringe. A separate syringe should be used for each product and care should be taken to inject each in separate places in the animal. Even if there is no apparent change in appearance when two drugs are mixed together, it does not necessarily mean that there has been no reaction between the two.

Where two or more drugs are being administered by mouth, they should also be administered separately. In particular, the product literature should also be consulted to make sure that there are no incompatibilities mentioned.

Where two or more drugs are being administered in the feed, again the product literature should be consulted to make sure that the drugs to be mixed are compatible.

If there is no statement in the literature and there is any doubt the manufacturers should be consulted.

The incompatbilities mentioned above relate to physical and chemical incompatabilities between the drugs. There can also be incompatability within the animal where one drug interferes with the elimination of a second drug. This may result in side effects. Once again, it is important that the product literature is read carefully before the drugs are given.

Conclusion
By following the manufacturers' instructions and exercising a little care it is possible to ensure that antibiotic preparations retain their potency for the duration of their stated live. The careful handling and administration of these preparations will minimise any long term risks to the user and will provide the patient with the intended dose of the active ingredient.

Note
[1] Definition as stated in the Report of the Joint Committee on the Use of Antibiotics in Animal Husbandry and Veterinary Medicine - November 1969.

Acknowledgement
The original author of the chapter acknowledges the advice given by Dr G Lukas, Ciba Geigy, Basle during the revision of this chapter.

Chapter 10

Vaccines

A S H Miller revised by Gillian Cowan

Unlike antibiotics, which may be given either to treat or attempt to prevent an infectious disease, vaccines are designed only for prevention. The effect of a vaccine - namely the induction of protection against a specific disease - is called immunisation.

Vaccines are generally prepared from micro organisms (most commonly live or inactivated viruses or bacteria as whole cultures, cells or extracts or a mixture of these) which stimulate an animal to develop its own specific immunity against the associated disease. Those parts of the vaccine to which the animal's immune system responds are called antigens. The micro organisms in the vaccine have been treated in some way - killed (inactivated), weakened (attenuated), or perhaps purified into specific antigens - rendering them safe to administer and unable to cause disease or ill-effects.

The process of immunisation depends upon an active response to the administered antigens. Thus, in order to ensure optimum results, the vaccine must be in perfect condition when delivered to the animal, and the animal itself should be as healthy as possible.

It is unfortunately true that immunity, even when established, has a delicate nature that can be compromised later by factors such as nutritional deficiencies, intercurrent infection or parasitism. Consequently vaccination should not be regarded as a panacea; the vaccine will raise the animal's resistance to the disease, but vaccination should also be accompanied by good animal husbandry to maintain the stock in healthy condition and to reduce the possibility of an overwhelming challenge by disease.

Shelf Life

In common with other pharmaceutical products, vaccines do not have an indefinite shelf life. Once the vaccine has been manufactured, its components begin a steady, irreversible loss of antigenic activity (or potency). This loss is normally very slow, but it can be hastened by incorrect storage conditions.

After delivery by the manufacturer the vaccine will maintain at least its minimum specified potency up to the expiry date printed on the container if stored under the recommended conditions. Different types of vaccine have differing shelf lives, so each expiry date should be noted. To obtain the authorised shelf life the manufacturer has had to generate data to prove that batches of the vaccine stored under the recommended conditions are still potent just beyond the quoted shelf life. He cannot predict potency, however, if a vaccine has not been stored under the recommended conditions.

Storage
It is impossible in the space available to give specific advice about the storage of all vaccines. The manufacturers' recommendations should always be followed: they will usually be found on the container, data sheet or package insert.

Some vaccines can safely be stored at room temperature, although extremes of heat (for example in kitchens, or on shelves over radiators) should be avoided. Other vaccines require refrigeration during storage: the temperature range often quoted is $+2^0$C - $+8^0$C. The exact temperature is not critical, but frequent fluctuations can be harmful.

It is advisable to place a maximum/minimum thermometer in the refrigerator where vaccines are stored. The thermometer should be checked and reset daily, to avoid incorrect storage. That the refrigerator should be set aside specifically for this purpose is preferable, to avoid the risk of contamination by other contents.

Vaccines should on no account be allowed to freeze, unless this is recommended by the manufacturer. Many vaccines suffer a considerable loss of potency and damage to the vacuum seal of the bung if frozen. Also, the adjuvant used in some vaccines will be damaged by freezing and render the vaccine non potent. If freezing occurs the vaccine should be discarded and replaced.

Transport
It is often necessary to transport vaccines to branch surgeries, farms or kennels. Most vaccines can travel in a car for a few hours without measurable loss of potency. If vaccines are being transported on a regular basis, a vacuum flask or freezer box may be a worthwhile investment. The container may be pre-cooled but, to avoid freezing the vaccine, ice or freezer packs should not be used. However, whether insulated or not, vaccines should not be left for long in a car on a hot sunny day - the temperature inside can rise to 40^0C (over 100^0F).

If the required number of doses is known, only that number should be taken. Vaccines not needed for immediate use should be refrigerated as soon as they reach their destination. If for any reason vaccine has to be returned to the main surgery or dispensary it should be plainly marked 'returned' and used as soon as possible thereafter. If should be remembered that vaccine suppliers cannot take back for resale vaccines which have been out of their premises for more than a few days as they cannot assure themselves that the vaccines have been stored correctly whilst out of their control.

Selection of patients for vaccination
As previously indicated vaccination will give the best results only if the animal is in a healthy condition when receiving the vaccine. The routine maintenance of animal health is outside the scope of this booklet but, briefly, the animal should ideally be free of the clinical signs of infectious disease, and should not show signs of severe parasitism or nutritional deficiency.

An individual examination of each animal is not always practicable, particularly when dealing with large groups of cattle, sheep or poultry. Also with such groups it is not always possible to choose a time when all the animals are perfectly healthy. However, wisdom may dictate that the whole group should be vaccinated, for the better good of all, if no disease sign is obvious. The vaccine manufacturer may be able to advise whether vaccination is inadvisable if a particular disease or condition is present. The manufacturer or veterinary surgeon may also indicate whether other procedures are permissible (for example dosing for worms) concurrently with vaccination.

In the case of pet animals a detailed examination is possible before vaccination. A small temperature rise may indicate only fear or excitement, but a larger rise may indicate disease and the wise course is to delay vaccination and re-examine the animal 24 hours later before deciding to proceed. (A small temperature rise a few days after vaccination is normal when certain live vaccines are used).

Vaccination is rarely effective in preventing disease in a farm or pet animals if it is already incubating the infection. Moreover, even the healthy animal may not become immune until several weeks after it has been vaccinated, and so measures should be taken to avoid exposure to disease during that time. For example, puppies should not be allowed into public places, and farm animals should not be allowed contact with other (possibly infected) stock, or with infected buildings or pasture, until immunity has become established - the manufacturer may have a specific recommendation. With many vaccines indeed, more than one dose is required to induce immunity; the first is a sensitising dose and immunity does not appear until after the second dose has been given. Consequently the above advice refers to the completion of a vaccination course.

Animals under the recommended age should not be vaccinated. Some vaccines are ineffective in very young animals because of the presence of maternally derived passive immunity. If there is any doubt the dose should be repeated when the animal is older.

The technique of vaccination

Vaccines may be given by many injection routes - intramuscular, subcutaneous, or intraperitoneal - as well as orally, or by surface routes such as the eye or nose. In all cases the advice of the manufacturer should be followed, so as to obtain the best results. With subcutaneous vaccines the manufacturer may recommend a particular site (for example behind the ear, in the scruff of the neck, over the ribs, or in the flank). The site is important not only to ensure a satisfactory level of immunity, but also in some instances to reduce the possibility or importance of local reaction. Vaccines should never be given intravenously, unless this is specifically recommended. Always read and follow the instructions given in the pack leaflet.

Killed vaccines are usually in liquid form ready to use. Live vaccines are often supplied in a freeze-dried state and require reconstitution with a sterile liquid diluent (or with a liquid vaccine if such combination is advised in the product information). Reconstituted vaccine should be used immediately and not stored.

Contamination

The site chosen for the injection should be free from signs of obvious contamination. In horses the common practice is to sterilise the injection site with surgical spirit, but in farm animals the result rarely justifies the means, and surgical spirit may even be contra-indicated when using certain live vaccines.

Sometimes vaccines are supplied pre-loaded into syringe or multi-dose injection packs. But when, in other instances, repeated doses must be withdrawn from the same container into a syringe, the correct technique must be observed to avoid contamination of the vaccine in the bottle. Often a needle is left in the bung and the syringe is attached when necessary. A different needle is then used to inject the animal - if the needle is dropped or becomes obviously contaminated, it should be discarded immediately. Note too that some vaccines must be shaken before any is withdrawn. Partly used packs should never be kept for long periods, and some may need to be discarded immediately. The manufacturer's advice should be followed carefully. Some vaccines may be used with automatic vaccination equipment. This is particularly recommended where no preservative is included in the vaccine which is intended to be used in a number of animals during one vaccinating operation. In the future, vaccine packs will carry warnings indicating the 'in use shelf life' of the product, ie the time between the withdrawal of the first and last dose of vaccine from the bottle. After this time, the container must be discarded.

Safety
Allergic reactions are possible, although rare, following the use of any injectable substances. They are mostly mild and pass off without treatment. However, in the unlikely event of a severe reaction, such as a swelling around the head and neck, difficulty in breathing or even collapse, veterinary attention should be sought immediately. Administration of antihistamine, corticosteriod or even adrenalin injections may be necessary depending on the type and severity of the reaction.

Overdosage with vaccines is uncommon, and rarely harmful except for the possibility of a local reaction. Vaccines intended for oral, intranasal or intra-ocular use should never be injected. With cats, droplets or injectable live vaccine should never be left on the skin where they can be licked off and swallowed. When, with any live vaccine, air bubbles are expelled from the syringe, care should be taken to ensure that aerosol droplets of vaccine are not released.

Unless there is a compelling reason or known precedent, vaccines should not be used in species other than those for which they are intended as both the beneficial and the side effects may be quite unpredictable.

Accidental Injection
The safety of the operators handling the animals and administering the vaccine is of great importance. Certain living vaccines, for example ovine contagious pustular dermatitis (orf) vaccine, are harmful if inadvertently injected into man or even if they come into contact with the human eye, mouth or grazed skin. Some vaccines, particularly inactivated ones, contain adjuvants which enhance the activity of the vaccine in the recipient animal. Some adjuvants are completely safe although they may cause harmless transient local reaction at the injection site. Some vaccines contain oil adjuvants which can cause severe local reactions if accidentally injected into humans. **If such an event occurs the site should be washed to remove excess vaccine and medical attention should be sought immediately. The vaccine pack should be retained and shown to the doctor.**

Mass vaccination of poultry
Because of the special needs of the poultry industry some live vaccines are given in the drinking water or by spray. Although such methods cannot

guarantee individual protection for each bird these procedures achieve a level of immunity which is sufficient to prevent the spread of disease. They offer a considerable saving in terms of labour costs, and a likely reduction in stress to the birds.

The recommendations of the vaccine manufacturer must be followed precisely. For example the containers used must be clean and free from rust and traces of disinfectant. The water used must be uncontaminated. The reconstituted vaccine must be used immediately and any unused material must be destroyed with an approved disinfectant thereafter. Special measures may be required for the protection of the operator: the literature supplied with the vaccine should be studied carefully before such vaccines are used.

Helminth vaccines
The only vaccines currently available in the United Kingdom for vaccination against disease caused by worms are those against husk (hoose) due to the bovine lungworm, *Dictyocaulus viviparus*.

They are oral vaccines and must not be given by any other route. The manufacturers provide specific and detailed advice on both storage and administration which should be followed precisely.

Vaccination in the face of disease
Sometimes it is necessary to vaccine groups of farm stock in which some animals are already infected. In such circumstances the complete protection of every animal cannot be achieved. Yet vaccination is worthwhile because it reduces the overall incidence or severity of the disease in the group.

Similarly, the vaccination of dogs against canine distemper is common practice as soon as they arrive at a rescue kennel or other infected premises. Although some of the dogs may already be infected at the time of vaccination and consequently will not be protected, the rapid protection given to others by the vaccination has been shown to result in a useful reduction in the disease incidence in the kennels and vaccination is therefore considered to be worthwhile. As the subsequent immunity of individual dogs is not certain, each must be revaccinated as soon as it is housed in a new home.

Chapter 11

Antiparasitic Products

Peter D G Bowen

Antiparasitics used for the treatment of animals are classified as ectoparasiticides or endoparasiticides depending on whether they are to control external or internal parasites. Now, however, there are endectocides which control both external and internal parasites.

Ectoparasiticides - as animal medicines, these are formulated as eartags, collars, dusting powders, shampoos, dips, pour-ons, aerosols and other sprays, for application to a wide range of domestic animals including horses, cattle, sheep, pigs, dogs, cats and other pets.

Endoparasiticides - these include anthelmintics for the control of roundworms, tapeworms, lungworms and liver fluke. They are administered as drenches, pastes, pills, feed additives, injections and even pour-ons. Also included are the antiprotozoals (eg coccidiostats) which are usually feed additives, but also soluble powders for inclusion to drinking water, in addition to injectables.

Endectocides - these may be used to control gastro-intestinal worms as well as lice, ticks and mange mites, in many domestic species of animal. In cattle they can also be used to control fluke, eyeworms and warbles; in sheep, nasal bots and scab; in horses, oral and gastric bots.

The safe storage and handling of the above basic classes of antiparasiticides are very different.

A.   ECTOPARASITICIDES

These products have in the past been based on organophosphorus compounds, or other cholinesterase inhibitors, many still are. Octopamine inhibitors can also now be used on some species of animals. There are also products derived from plants, like derris (rotenone) and pyrethrum (pyrethrins); more recently the synthetic pyrethroids and now insect growth regulators have been developed.

Pet Products
Products for pets, although they may contain the same active ingredients as farm products are, by virtue of their design and low concentration, safe for

use by members of the public with minimal precautions. **The advice on use, storage and disposal given in the label on pack leaflet should, nevertheless, be followed implicitly.**

Farm Products

Generally many insecticides, tickicides and acaricides (miticides) are potentially more toxic and hazardous than other medicinal products. This is because they are often concentrated, complicated to apply, and of necessity, as persistent as acceptably possible, with a concern for efficacy versus residues.

Storage

The requirements for storage and transit of farm products, often in large containers, are complicated by the need to consider the leakage of dangerous chemicals. All these substances must be treated with respect, including observance of the Control of Substances Hazardous to Health Regulations (COSHH) 1994 and Chemicals (Hazards Information and Packing) Regulations, 1994 (CHIP 2).

All such products should be stored in a dry, ventilated and well lit store in their original containers, tightly closed and in a safe place away from food, drink and animal feeding stuffs. The store should be locked against unauthorised persons, particularly children. Depending on the types and quantities of substances kept, the store will range from a simple cupboard, to a substantial purpose built structure designed as far as possible to contain products in the event of emergency such as fire. Guidance can be obtained from HSE leaflet AS18 or CS19 HSE Guidance note for farmers and other professional users on storage of approved pesticides and ADAS leaflet 767. The Code of Practice for the safe use of Veterinary Medicines on Farms should also be referred to. (See chapter 13).

Stores for dips and other pesticides should be situated in areas free from flooding and well away from drains, watercourses, ponds, sources of supply and groundwater catchment areas.
The floors within the store should:

* Be impervious to chemical penetration;
* Be easy to clean;
* Have a liquid-proof skirting extending above the damp course in the walls;
* Contain no internal drains connecting to sewer systems.

Store products above the level of the damp course to permit routine floor cleaning, and to avoid contaminating water should there be a fire.

External doors should have raised sills to prevent liquid draining from the building. If necessary the door-way should be ramped to allow vehicle access.

Drainpipes from the roof should be external but if internal they must be protected from physical damage and sealed into the floor.

Regular checks for leaking packs should be made.

Some products are flammable and this needs to be considered in storage.

Absorbent, non-combustible material to clean up spills must be readily available and clearly labelled, eg sand, sawdust or Fullers Earth.

Labels will always indicate the storage requirements for the avoidance of such hazards. In addition, requirements of the Medicines Act (1968), such as precautions to maintain stability and potency by protection from heat or cold, are given.

Handling
This includes not only using or applying the products but also the disposal of empty and damaged containers.

It should be noted that assessing hazards, reducing risks and taking precautions when handling sheep dips and chemicals are legal requirements under COSHH regulations.

All dip products and most ectoparasiticides contain hazardous substances. If mishandled, they can make you or animals ill and may pollute the environment. The harm products can cause depends on what active ingredient they contain (see the label) and how the products are applied.

Personal Protective Equipment (PPE)
For most ectoparasitic products operators should wear PPE as recommended by the manufacturer on the product package label or leaflet. Further guidance can also be obtained from the joint VMD/HSE/DoE leaflet 'Sheep Dips' AS29.

Remember:
* PPE should be servicable, clean and a good fit;
* Concentrated product can get through protective gloves and clothing. Wash it off PPE immediately;
* If you get a lot of contamination on your skin, PPE or personal clothing, wash your skin and put on clean clothes and PPE;

* Remove and replace damaged PPE such as cracked gloves, waterproof clothing with tears or which cannot be fastened properly, and leaking wellingtons;
* Wear the trouser/leggings over the boots. In general wear the sleeves of waterproof suits over the gloves and overall sleeves inside the gloves;
* Avoid handling animals still wet from treatment.

Record Keeping

Under COSHH, following the use or disposal of hazardous products a register should be kept containing:

(i) The names and addresses of all workers carrying out the handling of hazardous products.
(ii) The total numbers of hours worked and the dates.
(iii) Details of substances used and for what purposes.
(iv) A record of sickness and absences from work, possibly resulting from the operation.

Operator training

Whatever treatment is used, all operators must be adequately trained. They must be told about the risks involved, the precautions to take and the symptoms of ill health associated with the use of particular products.

It is now illegal to sell Organophosphate (OP) sheep dips unless the buyer has the support of a certificate[1]. Since 1 April 1995, anybody who buys OP sheep dip must have a Certificate of Competence in the Safe Use of Sheep Dips or satisfy the distributor selling the dip that they are the employer of, or acting on behalf of, somebody who has the certificate. This certificate shows that holders have passed a test of their knowledge of practical safety techniques.

The distributor will check that the person buying either shows a certificate or can give its number.

Read the Label

The warnings and precautions for ectoparasitic product use vary for different products depending not only on their active ingredients and formulations but also according to the way that they are applied and the animals to be treated. All the information is to be found on product labels and leaflets. Such label instructions should be followed **implicitly** to ensure the safe and efficient use of the product.

B.   **ENDOPARASITICIDES (anthelmintics; wormers)**

In contrast to the ectoparasiticides these products are relatively non-toxic, except at gross overdosage, and are very simply administered as small doses of undiluted product. These preparations are much less likely to contaminate the environment or constitute a hazard to operators. Nevertheless anthelmintics marketed more recently for farm use have labelling requirements on handling, etc that are becoming more and more comprehensive. For instance, levamisole products can cause side effects in some people so the warnings in data sheets should be carefully followed.

For the treatment to be successful, farm animals need to be dosed strategically with anthelmintics. A wide variety of products are marketed.

Parasite species treated
The term 'helminth' relates to internal worm parasite but individual products do not necessarily treat all the different types of these parasites, eg gut and stomach roundworms, lungworms, tapeworms and liver flukes. It is essential to choose the right product for the task at hand. The veterinary profession is aware that resistance can develop to anthelmintic products and hence strategic worming programmes designed to rotate the efficient formulations have been devised. (See Appendix).

Storage
Modern anthelmintics are now very much safer than they used to be and storage requirements are generally standard. However, many suspensions however should not be frozen and require to be well shaken before use. As with ectoparasiticides and, indeed, all animal medicines - anthelmintics should be stored under lock and key, tightly sealed in their original containers, away from food, drink and animal feedingstuffs.

Protection of the environment is vitally important.

Handling
Mainly non-hazardous although skin contact should be avoided in most if not all cases. Used empty containers or the product should not be allowed to contaminate ponds, waterways or ditches but triple rinsed and disposed of safely such as burial away from water courses.

C.   **ENDECTOCIDES**

These products which are used to treat both internal and external parasites are based on ivermectin, and recently introduced dorametin, and moxidectin.

Storage
Requirements are standard including protection from light.

Handling
Certain formulations may be irritating to human skin and eyes and therefore require personal protective equipment to be used (see label). Also operators should not smoke or eat while handling the product. With injectable formulations self injection should be avoided.

Very specific and different recommendations for disposal should be followed.

Appendix

Anthelmintic Resistance of Worms in Sheep and Goats: Practical help on avoidance.

The following text forms a leaflet produced in 1991 by the Central Veterinary Laboratory (CVL) (now part of the Veterinary Laboratories Agency) and NOAH, endorsed by the Sheep Veterinary Society, Moredun Research Institute, National Sheep Association and AHDA (Animal Health Distributors Association). Some slight changes have been made for clarification.

The problem: Worms (nematodes/round worms) are major parasites of sheep and goats and are controlled with anthelmintics (wormers/drenches). Anthelmintics are particularly important in lowland and intensive flocks to maintain high efficiency of production and animal welfare. Unfortunately it is in such flocks that resistance is most likely to occur.

Widespread resistance has already developed in Australia, New Zealand and South Africa to levamisole and benzimidazole anthelmintics. In the UK benzimidazole (white drench) resistance has been confirmed in the stomach worms *Haemonchus contortus* and *Ostertagia circumcincta* and in the small intestinal worms *Cooperia curticei* and *Trichostrongylus colubriformis*. Resistance has also developed to ivermectin on an experimental goat farm.

Once you have resistant worms on your farm for all practical purposes they are present indefinitely.

We cannot expect many new types of anthelmintics in the future so we must use correctly those that are available.

Despite many brand names, currently only three types of broad spectrum ANTHELMINTIC FAMILIES are available in the UK; Benzimidazoles,

Levamisole, Avermectins.

In addition, certain narrow spectrum anthelmintics are available that will control Haemonchus, an important blood sucking species.

The advice:
What you need to do.....

The following advice is designed to help you keep these anthelmintics effective on your farm.

Most important....
1. Work out a control strategy. Discuss with your vet the best strategy to control worms on your farm and in particular the use of grazing management.

You should also....
2. Avoid introducing resistant worms. Find out as much as you can about the history of the sheep/goats that you are purchasing including their history of anthelmintic treatments. Ensure all sheep/goats coming to your farm are dosed with an effective anthelmintic before arrival or upon arrival. If uncertain of which anthelmintic to use, give a combination of 2 or more of the anthelmintic families. Hold in a yard or pens for at least 24 hours after dosing before placing on pasture.

3. Use the correct dose. Check that your dosing gun is delivering the correct volume (use a plastic measuring cylinder for this).

   Do not guess weights. Divide sheep/goats into groups of similar size animals, weigh a few of the heaviest animals in each group and treat all the same rate as the heaviest in the group.

4. Do not dose unnecessarily. Work out a good worm control strategy with the help of your vet. The more often you treat your animals the more likely you are to select for resistance.

5. Change the anthelmintic family every year (not more often) prior to lambing. Resistance is more likely to develop if you stay with one anthelmintic family over an extended period. Remember there are only three anthelmintic families to choose from benzimidazoles, levamisole and avermectins. If in doubt consult your vet or registered distributor as to which anthelmintic family a particular product belongs.

6. <u>Check that your anthelmintic is effective</u>. Ask your vet to arrange a faecal egg count reduction test or a laboratory based test for you annually. If there is some resistance, continuing with that anthelmintic will only make matters worse.

7. Be aware that goats can transmit resistant strains of worms to sheep. Studies in New Zealand and the UK have shown resistant worms are more common in goats than sheep. So you are more likely to introduce problems into your sheep flock with goats. Do not keep sheep and goats together. Maintain separate sheep and goat pastures. Where goats are used for upland pasture improvement ensure they do not introduce resistant worms onto the farm. Remember, dose rates for goats may be different from those for sheep.

8. If resistance is diagnosed, in addition to the above:

    - Stop using the drench family to which resistance has been diagnosed. Seek veterinary advice.
    - Alternate annually between the remaining two drench families.
    - Check every year to ensure these are still effective. Consult your vet on the correct method.

To sum up:-

Do not buy-in resistant worms.
Give a quarantine drench.
Do not underdose by guessing animal weights.
Do not treat unnecessarily.
Do not change anthelmintic families more than once a year.
Do not use the same anthelmintic family year after year.
Do not use the same pastures for sheep and goats.
Do not mix different anthelmintics together yourself.
Do seek advice.

Notes
[1] SI No. 599/94 - The Medicines (Veterinary Drugs)(Pharmacy & Merchants List)(Amendment) Order 1994.

Chapter 12

Medicinal Feed Additives

David R Williams

Legislation was introduced in 1988 and 1989 under the Medicines Act to provide more stringent controls on the incorporation of medicinal products in animal feeds and on the sale and distribution of medicated feeds.

The Medicines (Medicated Animal Feeding Stuffs) Regulations 1988 came into force in two parts, the first in July 1988 and the second in July 1989. The major points of this legislation are as follows:-

medicated feed manufacturers, including on-farm mixers, have to register with the Royal Pharmaceutical Society of Great Britain who will enforce compliance (or Department of Agriculture in N. Ireland)

incorporation of medicinal additives is restricted to registered manufacturers or incorporators including home mixers

the sale, supply and importation of medicated feeds are restricted

a new standard form of Veterinary Written Direction (VWD) is introduced

feed manufacturers must comply with the relevant Codes of Practice, A or B, which cover quality, personnel, training, documentation, premises and equipment. The Codes of Practice are obtainable from MAFF Publications, London SE99 7TP.

The Regulations prohibit a person, in the course of a business carried on by him, from incorporating a medicinal product in an animal feeding stuff unless it is incorporated in accordance with a Marketing Authorisation (Product Licence), an Animal Test Certificate or a Veterinary Written Direction given by a veterinary surgeon or veterinary practitioner. Additionally, these Regulations generally require the person incorporating the medicinal product to be registered in Part A of a Register ("the Register") kept by the person appointed as Registrar under section 1 of the Pharmacy Act or by the Department of Agriculture for Northern Ireland in respect of the premises where the medicinal product is incorporated, if the medicinal product is incorporated at a rate below 2 kilograms per tonne. In any other case he must generally be registered in either Part A or Part B of the Register. The

Regulations generally prohibit a person not registered in Part A of the Register from incorporating in an animal feeding stuff a medicinal product for which there is no Product Licence(marketing authorisation) or Animal Test Certificate relating to the incorporation of that product in an animal feeding stuff. A person registered in Part B may only incorporate a medicinal product at a rate of 2 kg or more per tonne. A person operating mobile mixing equipment may be registered in respect of the premises where that equipment is normally kept.

The Regulations prohibit a person, in the course of a business carried on by him, from selling or supplying any animal feeding stuff in which a medicinal product, not being a Prescription Only Medicine (that is to say a medicinal product which may be sold or supplied by retail only in accordance with prescription given by a veterinary surgeon or veterinary practitioner), has been incorporated, or from importing any such animal feeding stuff unless the medicinal product was incorporated in the animal feeding stuff in accordance with a Product Licence, an Animal Test Certificate or a Veterinary Written Direction.

A second set of Regulations, The Medicines (Exemptions from Restrictions on the Retail Sale or Supply of Veterinary Drugs) Order 1989, were brought into operation on 1 July 1989. The major points of this legislation are:-

only registered manufacturers can obtain medicinal feed additives and medicated feed supplements.

it allows merchants to sell or supply PML feed additives and supplements to registered manufacturers.

allows PL holders, specially authorised persons, Category A manufacturers and wholesale dealers to sell or supply PML and POM feed additives to certain categories of registered manufacturers.

it contains lists of PML and POM medicinal products and medicinal feed additives.

The third piece of legislation is The Medicines (Intermediate Medicated Feeding Stuffs) Order 1989. This Order came into force on 1st July, 1989 and its major features are that it:-

provides that all medicated feed supplements (including protein concentrates) are to be treated as medicinal products, ie require a Product Licence.

brings all medicated feed supplements (including protein concentrates) within the controls on sale and supply.

The fourth piece of legislation is The Medicines (Exemption from Licences) (Intermediate Medicated Feeding Stuffs) Order 1989. As with the previous Order, this legislation was brought into operation on 1st July, 1989.

It exempts from the requirement to have a Product Licence for any medicated feed supplement (or protein concentrate) which contains a licensed medicinal feed additive incorporated in accordance with its Product Licence.

Types of medicinal feed additives
Medicinal feed additives are included in feeding stuffs mainly for therapeutic or prophylactic purposes. The wide definition of 'medicinal purpose' under the Medicines Act 1968 includes not only the treatment or prevention of disease but any prevention or interference with the normal operation of a physiological function.

Additives therefore are included in feeding stuffs for a 'medicinal purpose' if they are used for any of the following:

1. Growth promotion.
2. The prevention of disease (eg Coccidiosis, Blackhead, Swine dysentery).
3. The improvement of carcass quality.
4. The therapeutic treatment of disease.

Veterinary Written Directions
The Medicines (Medicated Animal Feeding Stuffs) Regulations 1988 introduced a revised standard form of Veterinary Written Direction, the essential features of which are:-

One new section added to permit veterinarians to cope with emergencies. Veterinarians may authorise incorporation by unregistered manufacturers in emergencies.

Should a veterinary surgeon decide to invoke the emergency procedures, then the new section has to be filled in by the veterinary surgeon concerned. In so doing he will have to complete one or more of the following sub-sections:-

1. Reasons(s) for authorising incorporation at a rate below 2kg/tonne of final medicated feeding stuff by a manufacturer (including on-farm mixers)

not in Part A of either RPSGB's Register or DANI's Register.

2. Reason(s) for authorising incorporation at a rate of at least 2 kg/tonne of final medicated feeding stuff by a manufacturer not in RPSGB's Register.

As with the current Regulations, the VWD has to be completed in triplicate by the veterinary surgeon, and is valid for 30 days.

UK Restrictions on sale or supply

Under the Medicines Act 1968 there are three categories of medicinal products in relation to retail sale: those on the general sale list, those only available through pharmacies, and those only available on prescription. All medicinal feed additives come into the latter two categories but in order to maintain the customary trading arrangements which have been built up over many years special exemptions have been made which enable registered animal health distributors to sell, amongst other products, medicinal feed additives to farmers (see Chapter 1).

The exemptions also enable specially authorised persons, Register A feed manufacturers and dealers in bulk veterinary medicines to sell such veterinary products to feed compounders on A or B Registers for inclusion in animal feeding stuffs.

The veterinary medicinal products which may be sold in this way are listed in schedules to the exempting regulations.

Under regulations which came into operation in 1989[1], provisions have also been made to ensure that the intermediate medicated feedingstuffs (eg protein concentrates and supplements) can be distributed by agricultural merchants. They will have to be registered animal health distributors as at present who can also distribute POM and PML medicinal products, or a second category of agricultural merchant who would be able to sell POM and PML intermediate medicated feeds but not POM and PML medicinal products.

Storage and handling of medicinal feed additives

Medicinal feed additives may reach the feed manufacturer in a number of forms. He may for example, purchase either the licensed medicinal products, or a supplement or protein/vitamin/mineral concentrate containing the veterinary drug. The diluted forms can usually be handled without difficulty provided that the containers are adequately marked and stored in specifically allocated areas.

Licensed medicinal products for inclusion in feedstuffs are generally highly potent preparations and it is imperative that they should be dealt with in a responsible manner. They should be stored in clearly marked containers under clean dry conditions, and in an area reserved specifically for them. Different potencies of the same product should be stored away from one another to avoid confusion.

Upon receipt the containers should be carefully examined for correct labelling, identity, and potency against the quality and quantity ordered. Under the new registration schemes the Code of Practice sets standards which are enforced by the RPSGB Inspectors.

Unlicensed Medicinal Products
New regulations were introduced in 1994: The Medicines (Restrictions on the Administration of Veterinary Medicinal Products) Regulations 1994 (SI 1994/2987).

The Regulations prohibit the administration of unlicensed veterinary medicinal products to animals except for specified purposes such as medicinal tests or where the Medicines (Veterinary Medicinal Products) (Veterinary Surgeons from Other EEA States) Regulations 1994 apply (regulation 4) or in specified circumstances to avoid causing unacceptable suffering to an animal (regulation 5). Additional rules apply where unlicensed products are administered to food-producing animals (regulation 5(2)), but less restrictions are applied in the case of treatment of minor or exotic species which are non-food-producing (regulation 5(3)). The Regulations also lay down standard withdrawal periods for animals destined for human consumption.

The Regulations control the prescription by veterinarians of veterinary medicinal products of all legal categories for animals under their care. Their effect for both food-producing and companion animal is *inter alia* to establish in law the "**cascade**". When no authorised veterinary medicinal product exists for a condition in a particular species, and in order to avoid causing unacceptable suffering, veterinary surgeons exercising their clinical judgement may prescribe for one or a small number of animals under their care in accordance with the following sequence:

(i) a veterinary medicine authorised for use in another species, or for a different use in the same species ("off-label use");
(ii) a medicine authorised in the UK for human use;
(iii) a medicine to be made up at the time on a one-off basis by a veterinary surgeon or a properly authorised person.

Under (i) above, the off-label use of both a product authorised for a different species and of one licensed for a different condition in the same species would be acceptable. However, the latter might be preferred when treating food producing animals since the data sheet withdrawal period could be used if the dosage was the same as or less than recommended; where a higher dose rate is used, or the product is licensed only for different species, a withdrawal period applies of at least the minimum specified should be applied.

The requirements apply to both food-producing and companion animals. In addition, veterinarians treating food-producing animals under the cascade in accordance with (i)-(iii) above should:

> only use medicines whose pharmacologically active ingredient (ie those which must appear on the product label) are contained in a product already licensed for use in the UK in food-producing animals. This is to ensure that residue implications have been evaluated;

> apply minimum withdrawal periods, of at least:

> - 7 days for eggs and milk;
> - 28 days for meat from poultry and mammals; and
> - 500 degree days for meat from fish;

> record certain information and retain it for at least three years from the end of the calendar year to which it relates.

Residues in Animal Products

The Ministry of Agriculture (MAFF) conduct regular tests on foods of animal and poultry origin for residues of medicinal products. Results of the surveys are published in 'MAVIS' which is issued by the Veterinary Medicines Directorate. The records show that the administration of medicinal products to food producing animals by incorporation in compound feeds is safe and efficacious. The avoidance of cross contamination of feeds is of the utmost importance to prevent residues and strict codes and practices are operated by registered feed manufacturers to this end.

Notes

[1] The Medicines (Veterinary Drugs)(Pharmacy and Merchants' List)(No.2) Order 1989. SI No. 2318
The Medicines (Medicated Animal Feedingstuffs) Regulations 1989 SI No. 2320.
The Medicines (Exemptions from Licences)(Intermediate Medicated Feedingstuffs) Order 1989 SI No. 2325.
The Medicines (Intermediate Medicated Feedingstuffs) Order 1989 SI No. 2442.

Chapter 13

Use of Medicines on Farms

Roger R Cook

During 1985 MAFF, in conjunction with fourteen different UK livestock and veterinary organisations produced the 'Code of Practice for the Safe Use of Veterinary Medicines on Farms'. In so doing they recognised the important part which farmers have to play in ensuring that the medicines produced and distributed to very high standards also reach the animals in the best possible condition. Also the Code is designed to ensure that what the animal produces, whether meat, eggs, milk or honey, is free from harmful residues when it leaves the farm on its way to the consumer.

In addition to advice on medicines storage and use, the Code introduced for the first time, a requirement for farmers to keep records of the medicines used in the animals treated. In 1988 this requirement became law, since updated as SI 2843, the Animals, Meat and Meat Products (Examination for Residues and Maximum Residue Limits) Regulations 1991. From May 1993 these records have had to be completed within **72 hours** of administration of the medicines. The Code of Practice is given below. A record book suitable for use by farmers to meet their statutory obligations is available from NOAH or AHDA, Gable Court, 8 Parsons Hill, Hollesley, Woodbridge, Suffolk IP12 3RB. The information to be recorded is as follows;

> Name of veterinary medicine;
> Date of Use;
> Identity of animal/group treated;
> Number treated;
> Date treatment finished;
> Date withdrawal period ended;
> Total quantity of veterinary medicine used;
> Name of person who administered veterinary medicine.
> It is also useful to record the batch number

Keep records of medicines stored separate from the medicines store in case they are needed by the Fire Brigade or other emergency services.

Information on Withdrawal Periods is contained in the booklet 'Withdrawal Periods for Veterinary Products' available from NOAH. Always ensure you are using the most up to date information.

CODE OF PRACTICE

Source of Medicines
1. Obtain your medicines only from your veterinary surgeon, pharmacy or registered agricultural merchant. Sales from other sources may be illegal and the medicines may not be safe or effective.

Storage
2. Store your medicines correctly in accordance with the instructions on the label. Storage temperature is critical for some medicines, especially vaccines. Light can damage others. Make sure your medicines are stored securely, under lock and key where practicable. Keep out of the reach of children, animals, or anybody not supposed to handle the medicines.

Record Keeping
3. Keep a record to show:

   quantity of any particular medicine purchased and the date it was purchased;
   quantity used, date and the identify of the animals (groups or individuals) it was used on;
   for each individual animal or group of animals treated, the dates of the beginning and end of the withdrawal period if required.

   A suggested layout for this record is given in the Animal Medicines Record Book, available either from NOAH or AHDA.

   When your veterinary surgeon prescribes Prescription Only Medicines (POM), he may wish to specify the form of record to be kept. Keep the record safely for at least two years. Your veterinary surgeon may need to see it.

Administration of Medicines
4. You or a reliable member of your staff should be personally responsible for the recording, safeguarding and administration of medicines and for seeing that the withdrawal period is observed. Your veterinary surgeon will be able to help with training in administration of medicines and injections. Untrained persons should not administer or have responsibility for medicines except under supervision.

5. Read the instructions carefully before administering the medicine. It is important that the dose and method of administration are right. In particular, the route and site must be right for injections.

6. Check any warning statements and guidance given about how the medicine should NOT be used, in particular, whether it can be used with any other medicines being given to the animal. Check the expiry date on the label: do not use if past that date.

7. Use medicines only on animals recommended on the label or leaflet, unless you have been directed to do otherwise by your veterinary surgeon. The result of giving a medicine to an animal for which it is not recommended is unpredictable and can endanger the animal. You also run the risk of committing an offence under Section 58 (2)(b) of the Medicines Act 1968 unless you are acting under the direction of your veterinary surgeon.

8. Consult your veterinary surgeon for advice about medication for sick animals.

Withdrawal Times

9. **Be careful to observe any withdrawal period laid down for the particular medicine between the end of treatment and the slaughter of the animals or the taking of their or milk for human consumption. If the animals are sold before the end of any withdrawal period, it is important that you tell the purchaser and/or auctioneer or other dealer.**

10. **It is vital to avoid residues in meat or other livestock produce, so observe these precautions strictly.**

Disposal of unused medicines or containers

11. Dispose of unused medicines safely when treatment is finished. Do not hoard partly used medicines just in case they may be useful later.

Injections

12. If administration of the medicines involves single or multiple injections, the simple rules in Appendix 1 will help to reduce the risks of spreading infection.

Emergency Telephone Number

13. Keep handy a list of emergency telephone numbers:
    local doctor
    local hospital
    your veterinary surgeon

APPENDIX

(i) Injections
The following simple rules will help to reduce the risks of spreading infection when giving single or multiple injections.

a. Disposable needles and syringes should be used where possible; take care to dispose of them safely;
b. ensure that all other equipment (needles, syringes, tubing etc) is cleansed and sterilised* before and after use. During use ensure that all equipment is left on a clean surface;
c. if you are using a syringe which requires to be filled from the bottle between doses, use one sterile needle left in the bottle during use to fill the syringe and a separate needle to inject the animal;
d. in the case of an automatic refill syringe, if an air bleed is required to equalise pressure as the injection fluid is withdrawn, use a sterile needle for this purpose;
e. use a sterile needle for the injection, preferably using a fresh needle for each animal or at least changing it frequently (every 10 or 12 animals) and sterilising* it between animals.
f. make the injection through an area of clean, dry skin. Do not inject through wet or dirty skin (clearly, fish have to be excepted);
g. all partially used bottles of vaccines should be destroyed safely, as puncture of the rubber cap can result in the contamination of the remaining contents;
h. if the operator is accidentally injected, medical help should be sought immediately.

* Needles should be sterilised by boiling, immersing in surgical spirit, or washing in disinfectant recommended for instrument sterilisation. General purpose disinfectants are dangerous if injected.

(ii) Antibiotic Residues Avoidance in Milk
In 1994 NOAH, acting in conjunction with Veterinary Medicine Directorate, British Cattle Veterinary Association, British Veterinary Association, Dairy Trade Federation, Milk Marque and National Farmers Union, issued the following advice in the form a leaflet sent to all dairy farmers:

Practical Steps
1. When any antibiotic preparation is used, identify and mark animal(s) to be treated.
   If mastitis is being treated with intramammary preparations, then, for treatment identification purposes, quarters should also be marked.

(a) Adopt a farm system for marking treated animals and quarters, and make sure everyone knows what it is.
Write the system on the plasticised chart and keep it in the parlour next to the marking equipment where everyone can see it.

(b) Mark the cow to be treated, and where necessary the quarter, before you leave the parlour to collect the treatment. This avoids treating the wrong animal or quarter.

It is recommended that a spray marker be used to mark treated quarters.

2. Use product as directed.
   (a) Follow precisely the manufacturer's instructions/veterinary advice.
   (b) If you are using intramammary preparations, make sure you distinguish between dry cow and lactating cow products.
   (c) Store medicinal products correctly. Keep them in a special box or cupboard and away from the bulk tank.

3. Wash hands after use.
Avoid contamination of milk, animals and equipment with antibiotic.

4. Write treatment in the record book.
   (a) After treatment, make sure that the identity of the product used and the withdrawal period are recorded correctly.
   (b) Record the identity of the animal treated and the withdrawal period in the treatment record book on each treatment occasion.

5. Observe withdrawal periods.
Record the milking at which the milk can go back into the bulk tank after the last treatment.

Milk from all quarters should be withheld, irrespective of treatment regime.

6. Keep contaminated and clean milk separate.
   (a) Keep contaminated milk out of the general milking system. Use a separate line or a separate milking bucket/unit.
   (b) Milk treated cows last if possible.
   (c) Do not mix dry cows with the milking herd.
   (d) Take precautions with newly purchased cows.
   (e) If in any doubt contact your purchaser.

7. For further advice, consult your veterinary surgeon.

(iii) **Feed Additives and Withdrawal Periods**

In the late 1980's particular concerns over residues in pig meat were addressed in a leaflet 'Feed Safety First' sent to all pig farmers in a joint initiative from NOAH, British Pig Association (formerly the NPBA), UKASTA (United Kingdom Agricultural Supply Trade Association) and FAC (Federation of Agricultural Co-operatives) which warned:

"Failure to heed this advice will lead to prosecution of offenders and jeopardise the future of all those involved in pig production". The main principles, which are relevant to **all** users of medicated feed, were as follows:-

Medicinal Feed Additives

In practice it is the incorrect use of medicinal feed additives, which could lead to residues in meat. Producers must pay particular attention to their use to ensure this can never happen.

Medicinal Feed Additives include:-

-prophylactic drugs such as anthelmintics (wormers)
-prescription products ie therapeutic drugs such as sulphadimidine
-growth promoters

Medicinal Feed Additives are split into two categories - PML (Pharmacy and Merchants List) and POM (Prescription Only Medicines), and they all have a marketing authorisation (product licence) issued by MAFF. The product data sheet, which is available on demand, defines important details such as uses, dosage rates and any warnings (including necessary withdrawal periods) that must be followed for each category of animal. In some cases, it will also set out precautions for safe handling by the users.

Withdrawal Periods - Their Importance

To make sure that there are no residues in meat, three rules must be followed:

(i) Always adhere to the withdrawal period stated on the data sheet for the product, the feed label or the veterinary written direction (VWD) (data suggested that as little as 2mg/kg of sulphadimidine administered to pigs can cause residues above 0.1mg/kg if no withdrawal period is observed).

(ii) Never allow pigs destined for slaughter to have access to dung from pigs fed on POM medicated feed.

(iii) Only use licensed products and ensure that your feed manufacturer is a registered manufacturer of medicated feeds. He will then be following the Code of Practice which minimises the risks of cross contamination. If home mixing, ensure that you are registered and follow the Code of Practice.

Producer Check List:
- Remove medicated feed before slaughter according to the instructions on the label, or as directed by your vet.
- Do not allow pigs due for slaughter to have access to dung from pigs still eating medicated food. At time of withdrawal, as much dung as possible must be removed from their pen to prevent recycling.
- Do not allow non-medicated feed to be contaminated by medicated feed. Special care is required if home milling and mixing; it is good practice to prepare feed for young pigs immediately after medicated feed, so that any contamination has plenty of time to work its way through the system. Otherwise the equipment can be flushed by processing clean grain and storing it for use in the next medicated batch.
- Never use the same bulk bin for both medicated and non-medicated feeds.
- Adopt a policy of sensible cleaning of all feeding equipment, troughs etc, and watering systems to avoid cross contamination.
- Keep records and instruct staff and relief staff to ensure disciplines are carried out.
- Keep samples of feed to help trace any breakdowns in the system. The samples should be kept in a cool place, properly labelled and in moisture proof containers.

Summary

Stick to these rules, and consumers can then have complete confidence that the pigmeat they are eating is entirely free from all feed additive residues and continues to be a safe and wholesome part of their diets.

Chapter 14

Protection of the Consumer

Kevin N Woodward

In the European Union (EU), veterinary medicines are authorised under two distinct pieces of legislation. Those intended for therapeutic use or for the alteration of physiological function (eg synchronisation of oestrus) are dealt with under the so called Veterinary Medicines Directives, 81/851/EEC and 81/852/EEC and their amending Directives, while those intended for prophylaxis, growth promotion or for the control of coccidiosis, and which are added to feed, are dealt with under Directive 70/524/EEC. As if to underline the difference, the former are dealt with through the European Medicines Evaluation Agency (EMEA) based in Canary Wharf in London or through national authorities in the EU (depending on the type of application) and come under the auspices of Directive General III (DGIII) in the Commission in Brussels while the latter are the responsibility of DGVI.

Both groups of drugs must meet criteria of safety, quality and efficacy before they are authorised. These criteria are laid down in the corresponding legislation. Quality and efficacy are not the subject of this article and will not be discussed further here except to point out that pharmaceutical quality covers such areas as contaminants and stability. Contaminants, either from the production process or those which arise due to instability under certain conditions may be toxic and so this area, often referred to as quality related to safety, is extremely important in the overall safety evaluation.

Safety refers to safety to the animal, to the environment, to users of veterinary drugs and to the consumer who will eat products of animal origin which may contain residues of veterinary medicines. It is the latter which forms the basis of this article although much of the scientific data generated for this purpose is required for the assessment of user safety.

Therapeutic Drugs

The main approach
The prime tool for the protection of consumer health for therapeutic drugs is the maximum residue limit (MRL). MRLs were previously established by individual Member States in the EU but they are now set at Community level. They are established by the Committee for Veterinary Medicinal Products (CVMP) through its Working Group on the Safety of Residues. The

latter had been examining the toxicology and residues issues of veterinary medicines and establishing MRLs on an ad hoc basis for several years when, in 1990, an EC regulation, Regulation (EEC) No. 2377/90 was introduced which established MRLs on a Community-wide basis. This legislation has two major consequences for drugs covered by Directives 81/851 and 81/852/EEC. Firstly, from January 1st 1992, no new pharmacologically active substance may be introduced on to the markets of Member States unless there is an EU MRL. Secondly, existing substances are subject to a systematic evaluation so that MRLs can be established for these by 1997.

To achieve the Regulation's ends, pharmacologically active substances are placed into one of four Annexes in amending Regulations to the original 2377/90. These are:

Annex I - full MRL
Annex II - no MRL required
Annex III - provisional MRL pending further data and subject to an expiry date
Annex IV - use in food producing animals is considered unsafe on consumer grounds and no MRL can be established

In addition to serving as safe limits, MRLs also serve other, but related purposes. From the consumer safety view point, they form the basis for establishing withdrawal periods. Moreover, they also form the basis for residues surveillance serving as regulatory limits and finally, their establishment at EU and international level should serve to remove barriers to international trade in both animal produce and veterinary medicines.

The basis for MRLs

Two concepts lie behind the establishment of MRLs for veterinary drugs - the no-observed effect level (NOEL) and the acceptable daily intake (ADI).

The NOEL is usually taken as the dose from toxicological studies, or for antibiotics, from microbiological studies, below which adverse effects do not occur.

It is usually determined in the most sensitive species for the most sensitive effect. The ADI is calculated by dividing the NOEL by a suitable safety factor (SF) which is usually 100 (10 for animal-human variation x 10 for human-human variation) but its value can be greater depending on the type of effect and the quality of data package. Occasionally, it may be smaller (usually 10) if the NOEL is based on effects in humans.

Thus, ADI = $\dfrac{\text{NOEL mg/kg body weight}}{\text{SF (100)}}$

If this is multiplied by the widely accepted 'standard' adult weight of 60kg:

ADI = $\dfrac{\text{NOEL} \times 60 \text{ kg}}{\text{SF (100)}}$

then the value is derived in terms of mg/person.

The elaboration of MRL is more problematic as there is no straightforward calculation and there is a large iterative element. It depends on a number of factors including the ADI, food intake values, the consideration of the intakes of extreme consumers (eg infants who have a high intake of milk, certain ethnic groups) and on the residues depletion profile (and hence on the pharmacokinetics of the drug) in each type of animal under consideration.

As a result of the difficulties in establishing dietary intakes, a standard dietary package is used for the elaboration of MRLs in the EU. This is as follows:

muscle	300g
liver	100g
kidney	50g
fat	50g
milk	1500ml
eggs	100g
honey	20g

Knowing that the ADI must be spread over such a package and knowing the residues depletion profile, an MRL can then be elaborated. The MRL must also take into account analytical capabilities. It is futile establishing any type of limit if it cannot be monitored and this is particularly true of MRLs. Indeed, it is a requirement of the legislation that drug manufacturers must provide a suitable analytical method for routine monitoring when they submit their dossier applying for an MRL. Any method of analysis must have a limit of quantification well below the MRL to render it practicable under field conditions.

Data requirements

For applications for MRLs under Council Regulation No (EEC) 2377/90, the data requirements are set out in the Annex to one of the veterinary medicines Directives, 81/852/EEC as amended by Directive 92/18/EEC which updates and consolildates the original Directive. The general requirements for toxicity testing are:

> single dose
> repeated dose - 90 days
> reproductive effects
> embryotoxicity/fetotoxicity (including teratology)(two species)
> genotoxicity
> carcinogenicity
> immunotoxicity
> pharmacokinetic data
> pharmacodynamics
> observations in humans
> microbiological data (for antimicrobial substances)

Tests for carcinogenicity, which are extremely expensive, are normally only required for drugs with structures similar to those of known carcinogens, for drugs which have produced positive effects in genotoxicity studies, and for drugs which have produced suspicious effects in other, shorter term studies. All the studies must be carried out, where possible, to approved international guidelines (eg OECD) and must be conducted in accordance with the principles of Good Laboratory Practice (GLP).

Residues data include pharmacokinetic studies in farm animals and residues depletion data. These too must be conducted in accordance with Good Laboratory Practice. It is necessary to identify the target issue, ie that which is selected to monitor for residues in the animal and which usually, but not always, has the slowest residues depletion rate. The marker residues, the residue whose concentration and depletion is in a known relationship to total concentration, must also be identified. This is important as the depletion of the marker residue must be characteristic of residues of the drug, which may be comprised of the parent drug plus an array of metabolites. Hence, the marker residue is essential for economic and practicable monitoring of residues. Applicants for MRLs must specify and detail the accuracy and specificity of their analytical methods, and identify the limits of detection and quantification. To put it another way, they must be able to specify the applicability and practicability of the method.

Withdrawal periods and surveillance
One of the major uses of the MRL is in the establishment of the withdrawal period. This is the minimum period between drug administration and slaughter or the collection of milk or other animal produce for human consumption. In the UK, it is usually set at the time that the marker residue falls below the MRL in the target tissues in all animals in a group from a serial slaughter

residues depletion study. Some countries favour sophisticated statistical methods of analysis for residues depletion and the establishment of withdrawal periods but these tend to be heavily reliant on substantially more animals than the simpler methods of the type used by the UK with no greater guarantee that animal produce will be free from residues that exceed the MRL.

The other major purpose in setting MRLs, as described earlier, is for surveillance purposes. This is usually for drugs with an MRL, but it is also used for drugs where there is no MRL, for example where unauthorised drugs are used illegally, or where prohibited drugs are used. In the EU, surveillance is conducted under Directive 86/469/EEC under the auspices of DGVI and Member States must submit annually a National Plan to the European Commission setting out their surveillance programme for the forthcoming year. At the present time the UK examines annually some 40,000 tissue samples for the violation of MRLs or for the presence of residues of prohibited drugs, but the incidence of positive findings is extremely low. Currently, the Directive only applies to residues in red meat, but there are plans to extend it to poultry, fish and other meat.

Progress with MRLs

A number of MRLs have been established in the EU since the Regulation came into force. Some of these are provisional (Annex III) pending further data from producers, and there are a number in Annex I (full) and Annex II (no MRL required). There are also a few substances in Annex IV (effectively prohibited for use in food producing animals).

Although some MRLs are the same for each species for any particular drug, some are different and even very different. These differences reflect those in pharmacokinetics, particularly in tissue distribution between different species, and underline the importance of having specific data on each animal for which MRLs are required. For these reasons, MRLs are species specific.

Progress with MRLs has previously been relatively slow because of the frequent need to elucidate issues with the companies concerned. However, many of these issues have now been resolved and significant progress is now being made.

Drugs authorised under Directive 70/524/EEC

As mentioned in the introduction, these are dealt with under a separate system to the therapeutic drugs. They are, nevertheless, considered for safety, quality and efficacy using the same principles and philosophies. Unlike the therapeutic drugs, compounds examined under Directive 70/524/EEC are not subject to Regulation No (EEC) 2377/90, nor are they subject to residues monitoring under Directive 86/469/EEC. However, the MRL approach is being considered for this group of drugs.

Conclusions

In the EU, the safety aspects of veterinary medicinal products are rigorously assessed before authorisation in Member States can occur, and great efforts are underway to establish MRLs for existing substances although it is important to recognise that these have been evaluated at the national levels in individual countries and form the basis for the present withdrawal period. Once MRLs have been established, there is an extensive surveillance system in operation to ensure they are complied with through the correct implementation and observance of withdrawal periods. Substances not considered safe for the consumer will be removed from the market by being placed in Annex IV of the Regulation (EEC) No. 2377/90, followed by residues monitoring for violations. As a result of these efforts the consumer is protected from the effects of potentially harmful residues. Overall, all veterinary medicines must fulfil the stringent criteria of safety, quality and efficacy before authorisations are granted.

Chapter 15

Disposal of Animal Medicines

Roger R Cook

Disposal
From time to time, at all stages in the distribution chain, the need will arise to dispose of damaged, outdated or outmoded animal medicines, as well as used containers and packages, contaminated sharps, applicators and protective clothing. In every case consideration must be given to worker, public and environmental safety, and to the specific properties of the individual product, with suitable protective clothing worn where appropriate. The nature of the product and its possible bulk may cause difficulties. A thorough product knowledge is called for with professional judgement if the right action is to be taken.

(a) **Contaminated Waste**
Always study the product label, data sheet or (where applicable) Safety Data Sheet for advice before disposing of used primary containers, which are likely to be contaminated even when empty.

Statutory controls for the disposal of waste are contained in the Control of Pollution Act 1975. Pharmaceutical and veterinary preparations fall into a special category of waste that must be disposed of in accordance with the Control of Pollution (Special Waste) Regulations 1980. The regulations provide for records to be kept whenever a consignment of special waste is transferred to carriers, operators or local waste authorities though it is clear the regulations were not intended to be a burden on commercial operations which do not warrant the controls. A heavy responsibility rests with those required to make decisions particularly in the case of damaged products where a source of danger exists and prompt disposal is imperative.

Normal methods of flushing, incineration and local refuse collection may or may not be applicable. Distributors, veterinary practices, farmers and feed compounders should contact either manufacturers or the local waste authority (county councils) for advice, particularly where the disposal of larger quantities of animal medicines is envisaged.

Some county councils operate chemical collection services which are able to dispose of periodic consignments of special waste, including waste containing arsenic, for example.

Special requirements relate to the disposal of controlled drugs and parasiticides which are dealt with in chapter 2 and 11 respectively.

(b) **Clean Packaging Waste**

In 1994 the Packaging and Packaging Waste Directive became European law, however at the time of writing (October 1995) it is not yet translated in to UK law, nor have the promised special measures for pharmaceutical packaging been produced by the EU Commission - we can only advise readers to be alert to any future imposition which could affect the disposal of outer packaging, such as transport cartons.

Disposal of Ectoparasiticides

The disposal of ectoparasiticides and in particular sheep dips, presents the greatest challenge and hence the need for care. Many ectoparasiticides can present potential hazards to operators, as well as to wild life and the public. The volumes involved tend to be greater, magnifying the problem.

Disposal operations should be regarded as seriously as actual use, with protective clothing and other precautions being utilised according to the manufacturers' instructions.

'Disposal' concerns not only leaking, damaged, and used containers, but also contaminated protective clothing and equipment, as well as waste diluted product such as dipwash remaining in a bath or other reservoir/applicator. Very generalised instructions as to disposal are indicated on labels, eg 'Wash out containers and dispose of safely' but refer also to the MAFF Code of Good Agricultural Practice for the Protection of Water (see further reading).

(a) **Empty containers**

Before the disposal of any container it must be thoroughly emptied. Where appropriate, containers should be rinsed into the spray or dip bath; and appropriate protective clothing worn as indicated on the product label. The container should be filled to about one quarter full with water, the stopper replaced tightly and well shaken. The rinsing should then be added to the dip. The rinsing procedure should be repeated three times.

(b) **Empty container pound**

Once the container is empty, and if possible, rinsed, it should be stored in a separate area to await disposal. This should be an 'Empty container pound' - a well defined and marked area, preferably under cover, from which unauthorised people, especially children, stock and pets, are excluded.

(c) **Disposal of empty containers**

Some local authorities will collect empty containers provided they have been thoroughly emptied and where possible, rinsed out and punctured. If the local authority does not offer a suitable service, then the containers should either be buried under the strictly controlled conditions outlined below, or a waste disposal contractor engaged to remove them.

Metal and glass containers (but no aerosols) - After removing caps and lids, metal containers should be holed and flattened. Glass containers can be crushed in a sack. These should be buried immediately at least 450mm (18 in) deep in an isolated place away from ponds, watercourses and boreholes. This place should be marked and a record kept of the site.

On no account should used containers be burnt - not only could product fumes be given off, but burning plastic containers can themselves produce toxic fumes.

Aerosol containers - Empty aerosol containers should not be burnt or punctured, but can be placed in ordinary refuse bins, amongst other rubbish.

Disposal instructions on small containers for dusting powders, shampoos and ready-to-use ectoparasiticides for pet animals are relatively simple. The packaging (except for aerosols and glass) can be safely burnt, and the dilute nature of the products makes them generally of minimal hazard to the user. No significant residue or environmental pollution problems are posed.

Empty containers should always be disposed of, or destroyed so they cannot be re-used for other purposes thereafter.

(d) **Disposal of unwanted product**

If the container is in good condition, ie is unopened with the label intact, the supplier should be asked to collect it. When opened or partly empty containers are to be disposed of, the manufacturer, local authority or waste disposal contractor should be consulted.

(e) **Spent sheep dip**

Advice can be sought from the National Rivers Authority, the local Ministry agricultural adviser, or the manufacturer. Some products have instructions on how to breakdown the spent dip in-situ prior to disposal. The main aim is to ensure that water resources are not polluted. The regulations and recommendations are regularly reviewed and it is important to check that the latest advice is being followed.

The generally accepted method is to spread the liquid over a suitable level area of soil at the rate of approximately $1/2$ litre/m^2. This should ensure that there is no surface run-off and seepage to sewers, streams, watercourses, open waterways, ditches, fields under drainage. Dilution of 1 part dip by 3 parts or more of water or slurry may be necessary to achieve this application. The area should not be accessible to the public and livestock should be excluded for a period of one month. Alternatively, a reputable waste disposal contractor can be used.

Soakaways are no longer recommended for the disposal of used dipwash.

If there is not a suitable area of land on a farm the used dip should be stored in a suitable holding tank until it is collected by an approved waste disposal contractor. Details of local contractors can be obtained from the local Waste Disposal Authority.

Ectoparasiticite products for domestic animals should also be disposed of carefully, in accordance with manufacturers' instructions.

Notes

Examples of statutes that impinge on the storage, transportation and disposal of animal medicines are the Misuse of Drugs Act 1971, The Control of Pollution Act 1974 and the Health and Safety at Work, etc 1974.

The Control of Pollution (Special Waste) Regulations 1980 (SI 1980 No. 1709) were made under section 17 of the Control of Pollution Act 1974 to take account of obligations arising from EEC Directive 78/319 concerned with toxic and dangerous waste.

Reference can also be made to a circular from the Department of Environment (Circular 4/81 of 20 February) available from branches of HMSO, which is a guide to the interpretation of the regulations.

Reference is made to the Control of Pollution (Special Waste) Regulations 1980 (SI 1980 1709). Prescription only medicines, biocides and phytopharmaceutical preparations are among the substances listed in Schedule 1 to the regulations which are designated as 'Special Waste' and must be disposed of in accordance with the notification procedures specified in the regulations.

The regulations were not intended to be a burden on small operations which do not warrant the controls (Guidance note from the Department of the Environment, 4/81). It is now necessary to consult the National River Authority about consent for the disposal of spent dip.

Advice can also be sought from local authorities: agriculture departments, or the Department of the Environment.

Section 2(1) of the Food and Drugs Act (1955) also applies to Ectoparasiticides.

Appendix

References and Further Reading

NOAH Compendium of Data Sheets for Veterinary Products

The Royal College of Veterinary Surgeons - Legislation Affecting the Veterinary Profession in Great Britain

The Royal College of Veterinary Surgeons - Guide to Professional Conduct 1992

Dale and Appelbe - Pharmacy, Law and Ethics 5th Edition - The Pharmaceutical Press, London 1993

Margaret A Cooper - An Introduction to Animal Law, Academic Press 1987

The Veterinary Formulary ed.Y.Debuf 2nd edition 1994, Pharmaceutical Press, Royal Pharmaceutical Society of Great Britain

Medicines, Ethics and Practice: a guide for pharmacists No 14, April 1995

Code of Practice for the retail sale or supply of animal medicines by veterinary surgeons, BVA Publications, revised 1995

Code of Practice for the prescribing of medicinal prodcuts by veterinary surgeons, BVA Publications, revised 1995

British Pharmacopoeia (Veterinary) 1993 - addendum 1995

British Pharmacopoeia 1993 volumes I and II - addendum 1994; 1995

European Pharmacopoeia

MAFF (1985) Code of Practice for Merchants Selling or Supplying Veterinary Drugs - Ministry of Agriculture, Fisheries and Food, Alnwick

MAFF (1985) Code of Conduct for Saddlers Selling or Supplying Horse Wormers - Ministry of Agriculture, Fisheries and Food, Alnwick.

BVA/RCVS/ADAS (1986) The Veterinary Written Direction and Withdrawal Periods, British Veterinary Association, London; Royal College of Veterinary Surgeons, London

MAFF Environment Matters

Codes of Good Agricultural Practice for the Protection of Water, Soil and Air (available free of charge) from MAFF Publications, London SE99 7TP)

Legislation
Medicines Act 1968
Medicines Act 1971
Misuse of Drugs Act 1971 and the Misuse of Drugs Regulations 1985
Agriculture Act 1970
Health and Safety at Work, etc Act 1974
Animal Health and Welfare Act 1984

Further Information
Further guidance on recent developments in marketing authorisation procedures and related matters concerning veterinary medicines is available in other AMELIA guidance notes. The following are currently available:

AMELIA 1	-	Provisional Marketing Authorisations
AMELIA 2	-	An Introduction to the Marketing Authorisations for Veterinary Medicinal Products Regulations 1994
AMELIA 3	-	Marketing Authorisations for Veterinary Medicinal Products: Duties on Holders and Variation Procedures
AMELIA 4	-	Marketing Authorisations for Veterinary Medicinal Products: Requirements for Labels and Package Inserts
AMELIA 5	-	Applications for Marketing Authorisations for Veterinary Medicinal Products
AMELIA 6	-	Renewal of Marketing Authorisations for Veterinary Medicinal Products
AMELIA 7	-	How Veterinary Medicines May Be Made Available in the UK
AMELIA 8	-	The Medicines (Restrictions on the Administration of Veterinary Medicinal Products) Regulations 1994 - Guidance to the Veterinary Profession

Further information is available from the Veterinary Medicines Directorate, Woodham Lane, New Haw, Addlestone, Surrey KT15 3NB - Tel (+44)(01932 336911, or Fax (+44)(01932) 336618, as follows:

- on the detailed requirements of the Regulations, and the implications of EC law, please contact the VMD's European and Information Policy Branch on extension 3035.
- on applying for a marketing authorisation, please contact the VMD's Licensing Administration Branch on extension 3037.